T

⌐NEEDS ASSESSMENT STRATEGIES FOR HEALTH EDUCATION AND HEALTH PROMOTION

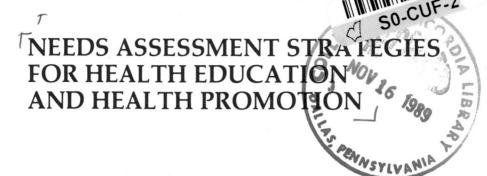

D1708683

A

Gary D. ⌐Gilmore⌐ M.P.H., Ph.D.
M. Donald Campbell, Ph.D.
University of Wisconsin
LaCrosse, Wisconsin
Barbara L. Becker
Wausau Family Practice Center

Benchmark Press, Inc.
Indianapolis, Indiana

Copyright © 1989, by Benchmark Press, Inc.

ALL RIGHTS RESERVED.

Reproduction or translation of any part of this work beyond that permitted by Sections 107 and 108 United States Copyright Act without the permission of the copyright owner is unlawful. Requests for permission should be addressed to Publisher, Benchmark Press, Inc., 8435 Keystone Crossing, Suite 175, Indianapolis, IN 46240.

Library of Congress Cataloging in Publication Data:

GILMORE, GARY D. 1943–

NEEDS ASSESSMENT STRATEGIES FOR HEALTH EDUCATION AND HEALTH PROMOTION

Cover Design: Gary Schmitt

Copy Editor: Lynn Hendershot

Library of Congress Catalog Card number: 87-72235

ISBN: 0-936157-24-0

Printed in the United States of America
10 9 8 7 6 5 4 3 2 1

The Publisher and Author disclaim responsibility for any adverse effects or consequences from the misapplication or injudicious use of the information contained within this text.

Dedication

For John and Ruth; Elizabeth, Scott, Todd, and Merrily, for being there.
For Louise, David, and Andrew.
For Marty, wise and trusted friend.

120416

Contents

Preface

The interest in, and use of, needs assessment strategies for health education and health promotion is accelerating. More individuals with these responsibilities are being called upon to start or continue planning efforts based upon the assessed needs of the populations they serve. Though structured needs assessment procedures have been used in health education to some degree for the past three decades, their use has been accelerated by a variety of factors: an increased desire to be as cost-effective as possible; increased emphasis on using marketing strategies which encourages segmentation of target populations based upon inherent demographic factors and special needs; a focus on accountability for the actions one takes as a health professional; and the upsurge of consumers who have bought into the health promotional bottom line of assuming more responsibility for their own well-being, thus becoming more willing to assess and address their needs.

We began this effort based on our involvement in health-related planning and the perceived need to clarify and organize individual and group needs assessment strategies. We did not intend to develop an all-inclusive document, rather one that would address established strategies. We also believed there were certain strategies which actually were needs assessments, but had not been fully recognized as such (for example, General Health Status Inventories for self-assessment). It was our intention to categorize the available strategies, review them, and provide examples of their use, based upon our experiences and those of others. Additionally, we wanted to offer examples of various combinations of strategies used in a variety of settings through the expanded discussions in the case studies. These provide an overview of the settings, specific target audiences, approaches to assessing needs, and the handling of any problems encountered along the way. Inventory examples are included so they may be considered for use in your assessment designs.

Overall, we wanted this to be a practical handbook which would have direct use in health education and health promotion planning and program development efforts. We have kept it as reader friendly as possible, and hope that it will become a well-worn resource for the professional.

We would like to acknowledge those who have assisted us in the development of this book. These people have provided insight, experiences, resources, and critiques which have enhanced the final product: Nancy Baumgarner, Val Chilsen, Gerald Matheson, Jay Schindler, Deborah Thalacker, and Dorothy Wetterlin. Additionally, we recognize

Martha Alexander, Charles Althafer, Claudia Bannon, Ruth Corcoran, Jack Curtis, Allan Erickson, Nancy Freeman, Jessie Gruman, Robert Harris, Robert Jecklin, Lauve Metcalfe, and Susan Wabaunsee.

Gary D. Gilmore
M. Donald Campbell
Barbara L. Becker

Part I

Introduction and Overview

In Chapters 1 and 2, we will present some of the key issues related to needs and needs assessments, and how they fit into the bigger frameworks of planning for health education and health promotion. Additionally, we will address the preliminary perspectives we formulate as health professionals through intuition, assumptions, secondary information, and experiences. We also present some of our basic premises, upon which the book is based.

1

Gaining a Needs Assessment Perspective

INTRODUCTION

Trends

Over the last 10 years, we have noted some changes regarding needs assessment. First, more health professionals appear to be using it as part of their work in hospitals, clinics, public health departments, voluntary agencies, private agencies, and business sites. This may be due to a great emphasis on documentation to justify program efforts and costs, as well as the increased use of marketing strategies in health-related settings. Also, cost-conscious consumers are becoming more selective in their health care choices, based to a large extent on a desire to have specific needs met at a reasonable cost. In response, health program and service providers have a renewed interest in ascertaining what some of these needs are, as revealed by the consumers. All of these aspects—documentation, marketing strategies, and program and service offerings—typically use needs assessment as a starting point for determining specific population needs, which in turn guide more effective planning and implementation strategies.

Second, there is a wide variance in what is meant by "needs assessment" and how it is used. There is much debate as to what a "need" is, whether or not we assess actual or perceived needs, and what the exact value of the needs assessment process is. Health professionals have different reasons for using this process. Some professionals use them as starting points for program planning. Others use them on a continuing basis with the same target audience to detect changing needs over a certain period of time, and to adjust the services based on those needs.

Third, while the first two considerations address group needs assessments, we have noted an emergence of individualized assessment strategies. These personal approaches can be quite valuable in health maintenance and health promotional efforts (see chapters 9 and 10). They can enable a person to detect specific risk factors which may negatively affect his or her health. Individualized assessment strategies also can help a person identify other factors which are quite positive and enhance good health.

Whether one is a health professional just beginning employment, or someone with considerable experience, the meaning and process of needs assessment can be quite unclear. The following is an example of a health professional who is taking on some new responsibilities. She is beginning to examine certain needs assessment possibilities and seeking clarification about their importance in her work.

A Case in Point

Lynn Dwier has worked as a public health educator for six years. She has been hired as the director of health education by a county health department in a midwestern state. Her primary responsibility is to serve as director of educational program development in primary prevention and health promotion. She supervises one other health educator. Together they are to develop public educational programs which focus on childhood and adult immunizations, the prevention and control of sexually-transmitted diseases and other communicable diseases, as well as general health enhancement. Additionally, Lynn has been asked to oversee staff in-service opportunities and to explore outreach options in local occupational settings. Lynn's in-service responsibilities include the development of staff training sessions in personal and professional health areas, such as stress management and communicable disease updates. Lynn's supervisor supports the development of new programs and services that will address the changing needs within her department and the community.

Lynn has reasoned that needs assessment could document those needs. However, she has some questions: What do we mean by a need? What do we mean by needs assessment? Are the reported needs actual or perceived?

Addressing the Questions: Lynn's questions are basic to an understanding of needs assessment and should be addressed individually.

What is a need? A need is the difference between the present situation and a more desirable one. The present situation may have some undesirable characteristics which motivate one to consider a more desirable situation. For example, we might realize that we are overweight and "need" to identify the causes and ways to resolve the problem. But needs are not solely related to undesirable situations; a very positive situation can be further enhanced. For example, one might jog two miles every other day to keep fit, and want to increase the distance. Or, one might have learned to avoid some of the risk factors related to cancer (e.g., smoking) and now wants to learn more about protective factors against cancer (e.g., adding more fiber to our diet).

What is a needs assessment? A needs assessment is a process which identifies the reported needs of an individual or a group. Individuals can conduct needs assessments which reveal reported areas of personal needs. A person can review these needs, consider their relative importance and practicality, and then take steps to address them. With groups, there can be representation by a smaller sub-group which is then taken through the needs assessment process. Health professionals can use the reported needs from this representative group for planning purposes.

Are the reported needs actual or perceived? It is difficult for the health professional, and even the target audience, to know if the needs identified by an individual or group are the actual needs (the *true* needs). These actual needs are difficult to identify and measure because they are continually changing. Perceived needs are those envisioned and reported by the participants in a needs assessment process. We refer to these as the reported needs. As health professionals involved in a needs assessment, we rely upon people as primary sources of information. These people draw from their experiences, observations, ideas, opinions, and feelings to guide them toward conclusions about needs—perceived needs. We recognize the importance of perceived needs because they represent the experiences and perceptions of the individuals or groups involved.

We believe it is inefficient to expend a great deal of energy trying to determine if perceived needs are actual needs. As individuals and groups are continually changing and growing, so are their needs. The focus of the strategies we present is not to determine true needs beyond any shadow of a doubt. Our purpose is to describe workable processes which assess issues of individual and group importance.

Why conduct a needs assessment? A needs assessment provides a logical starting point for individual action and program development, as well as a continuing process for keeping activities on track. As we will describe later in this book, needs assessment can be repeated to monitor program impacts. This process enables our educational and promotional efforts to be guided by a realistic data base. Overall, a needs assessment process can assist health professionals in a variety of ways: program development efforts can be based on reported needs; changes and trends can be assessed over a period of time; individuals and target audiences can be involved in purposeful activities; and the target audience can be more closely characterized.

BALANCING SCIENCE AND ART
Qualitative and Quantitative Issues

Human needs are diverse and changing. No single approach to assessing them would always be appropriate. A variety of approaches is necessary. One way to vary the approach is to consider both quantitative and qualitative information. Health professionals are familiar with quantitative data. Newspapers are full of statistics describing increases in health care costs, changes in the incidence of specific diseases, and various lifestyle trends. Professional journals rely heavily on quantitative data to report the results of scientific and applied research. Most people usually have a greater familiarity, and perhaps security, with numbers. Our society has been conditioned to accept something ranked number one, rather than number 20.

However, numbers do not tell the full story. In fact, they can over-simplify. They need to be balanced with qualitative data. Narrative information is necessary to elaborate on statistical data. A narrative format can capture variations and exceptions, and portray the needs as completely as possible.

For example, in Lynn Dwier's new employment situation, she may have to rely on a variety of qualitative and quantitative information sources in order to clarify the needs. Specifically, in Lynn's community, there is a high incidence of teenage deaths. Recent local statistics on the causes of teenage deaths show that motor vehicle accidents represent the leading cause of death. Other sources of information include Lynn's co-workers, her immediate supervisor, and key individuals in the community. Discussions with these people may indicate factors which contribute to motor vehicle accidents, such as alcohol consumption, failure to use seat belts, and stress in the family. This qualitative information yields a more complete picture of teenage deaths and suggests possible needs for Lynn to address.

Intuition

Our instincts and feelings count in needs assessment. In addition to gathering quantitative and qualitative information, these more intuitive responses of health professionals and community members are also important and should not be ignored.

As a psychological construct dealing with a certain preference for perceiving, Briggs Myers (1980) has provided insights into the intuitive focus. In contrast to perception through facts and details, intuition focuses on ideas and possibilities. She notes:

"when people consider their own mental processes, it will be evident that more than one kind of perception is possible. People are certainly not limited to the direct report of their senses. Through the subtle messages of intuition, people can also become aware of what might be or can be made to be." (p. 25)

Drawing from this orientation, Agor (1984) examines the value of intuition for making practical management decisions. He cites examples, as well as data from his own research, which demonstrate how some successful managers make major decisions based on intuition. In some cases, intuition takes precedence over conflicting or inadequate information. In a national study involving 1,679 managers, Agor found intuition more prevalent with those advanced in management rank. Top managers in every sample group tested used intuition in decision making to a greater extent than middle and lower managers.

Generally, intuition increases with experience. New health professionals may not have a wealth of experience on which to draw. There may be hesitation in trusting individual feelings about needs and priorities, and a desire to rely more extensively on quantitative data. With increasing experience, however, individual insights take on a greater significance in the planning process.

Assumptions and Assessments

Two groups are involved in a needs assessment. One group is comprised of the professionals directly involved in the planning, coordinating, or facilitating of the needs assessment. They bring to the process health-related expertise, and often previous needs assessment experience. The other group is the target audience or target group. These individuals bring their expectations and life experiences, which help them identify a range of needs, wants, and interests.

When the two groups enter into the needs assessment process, individuals in both groups bring some assumptions about what the needs are. These assumptions are intuitive in nature, influenced by the previous experiences, opinions, feelings, and ideas of each individual. The health professionals develop assumptions based on ongoing interaction with community members and other professionals, the examination of demographic data and vital statistics, the comprehension of the various political and socioeconomic forces influencing the community, and personal insights, awareness, and experience. Members of the target audience draw from their own insights and experiences in making their own needs assumptions.

If accurate, these needs assumptions can be very helpful in forming a starting point. They can help to narrow the focus of a too-broad or too-generalized approach to a needs assessment. They can help to start the assessment process in the right direction.

However, needs assumptions are not meant to take the place of a needs assessment. In a sense, they are precursors to a set of reported needs. It is through the needs assessment process that these assumptions become more clearly defined, and possibly revised, resulting in some specifically identified needs.

Once specific needs have been reported, it is important for the health professional to present the results of the needs assessment to the target audience. This presentation gives the target audience the opportunity to clarify and acknowledge the extent to which the identified needs accurately reflect the needs of the group. Then the health professional and target audience can reach a joint resolution regarding needs to address, and how best to address them.

SOME BASIC PREMISES

Our approach to needs assessment is based upon certain premises. Prior to your review of the individual and group needs assessment processes in the following chapters, consider these points:

1. *People* are important to the needs assessment process. Individuals have the capacity to reflect on their health-related needs and to report these needs. Practitioners also can draw from their education and experience to reflect and report on the health-related needs of the people with whom they work.
2. The *needs* that people report are realistic issues to consider, particularly when there is a trend. We can view reported needs as one source of information. (We will address other sources in the forthcoming chapters.)
3. A *needs assessment* is an applied process for gathering useful information for individual and group planning purposes. Its basic purpose is not to construct or test a scientific hypothesis, although good research techniques often are used in data collection and analysis.
4. *Planning committees* are important to the needs assessment process. Often, committees are established after the needs have been determined and the program is about to be planned. But, a planning committee also can help to plan and conduct a needs assessment. The committee can determine the kind of needs to consider, from whom to gather information, and what strategies to use. Committee members can also assist with data collection and analysis. Involving a planning committee at this early stage can ensure that the program is based on the perceived needs of the intended participants.
5. A *needs assessment is an integral part* of the program planning process. A needs assessment is one step toward planning effective health education and health promotion activities.

SUMMARY

We have had an opportunity in this chapter to address the increased focus on needs assessments, questions regarding their nature, some of the basic principles, and our own premises. Human needs, while complex, are able to be assessed within the context of target group settings and situations which impact on those needs. Health professionals also have a context from which to draw preliminary need-related inferences based upon experiences and impressions. However, these are only starting points for the professional; these are clues of possible target group needs. Health professionals must consider the value of determining in a structured fashion the prioritized needs of a target group, so that effective health educational and promotional efforts can be continued, adjusted, or newly-developed when appropriate.

2

Needs Assessment Within The Bigger Picture

INTRODUCTION

Needs assessment for health education and health promotion does not stand alone. It is part of a bigger picture of the development, implementation, and evaluation of health education strategies for health promotional purposes. In this chapter, you will have the opportunity to study key contexts for the needs assessment strategies detailed in later chapters. These include: the meaning of health promotion and health education, program development, the development of advisory and planning committees, preliminary observations, and needs prioritization.

THE CONTEXT OF HEALTH PROMOTION AND HEALTH EDUCATION

The terms health promotion and health education encompass broad dimensions in addressing health, a term which also has a variety of definitions. Though the World Health Organization's (WHO) definition of health moved us into a multidimensional understanding ("a state of complete physical, mental and social well-being and not merely the absence of disease or infirmity" (World Health Organization, 1985), it has been critiqued as more of an ideal than a reality which can be obtained (Noack, 1987).

Noack has offered a definition of health which is more process and systems oriented, and can be considered an operational definition of health: "A state of dynamic balance—or more appropriately as a process maintaining such a state—within any given subsystem, such as an organ, an individual, a social group, or a community" (Noack, 1987, p. 14). He adds that health has two key dimensions: health balance (a dynamic equilibrium), and health potential (capacity for equilibrium between person and environment), at the individual and community levels in both instances. Examples of health balance at the individual and community levels would be a relaxed state and a subjective sense of family well-being (assessed through indicators of health and quality of life), respectively. Examples of health potential at both levels would be good nutritional status and the proportion of a health agency's budget aligned with health promotion activities, respectively.

Health promotion can be viewed as a collective effort in attaining health. More specifically, it is defined by a WHO Working Group in Europe (1987) as the process of enabling people to increase control over, and to improve, their health. This promotional perspective is derived from a conception of health as the entent to which an individual or group is able to realize aspirations and satisfy needs, and to change or cope with the environment. Health in this context is seen as a "resource of everyday life, not the objective of living; it is a positive concept emphasizing social and personal resources as well as physical capacities" (p. 654). Basic aspects of health promotion cited by this group were enabling "people to take control over, and responsibility for, their health as an important component of everyday life—both as spontaneous and as organized action for health"; requiring "the close cooperation of sectors beyond the health services, reflecting the diversity of conditions that influence health"; combining "diverse, but complementary, methods or approaches, including communication, education, legislation, fiscal measures, organizational changes, community development and spontaneous local activities against health hazards"; encouraging "effective and concrete public participation" encompassing the development of individual and collective problem solving and decision making skills; and involving health professionals in education and health advocacy, particularly those in primary care (p. 654).

In attempting to achieve these aspects of health promotion, recommendations were advanced which focused on equitable health policies, work and home environments conducive to health, establishment of social networks, social support, coping strategies, and health-related lifestyles, along with increases in knowledge as drawn from epidemiology, social, and other sciences. With this as background, the Working Group cites a series of selected considerations for prioritizing health promotion policy development:

- indicators of health and their population distributions;
- current population knowledge, skills, and health practices;
- current policies in government and other sectors;
- expected impact on health;
- economic constraints and benefits;
- social and cultural acceptability; and
- political feasibility. (Working Group on Concepts and Principles, 1987, p. 657)

Health education is an educational context within health promotion. Though numerous definitions of health education exist, we have found that much of what is practiced relates to the blending of two widely recognized definitions. Green et al. (1980) define health education as "any combination of learning experiences designed to facilitate voluntary adaptation of behavior conducive to health," (p. 7); Ross and Mico (1980) specify that it is "an educationally oriented process of planned change which focuses on those behaviors or problems that directly or indirectly affect people's health" (p. 7). The former definition provides a broader scope for health education, particularly considering the diverse nature of health. The latter definition emphasizes the process of planned change, underscoring the approach of much health education activity today. The aspect of the health educator planning educational experiences which foster health enhancement voluntarily is a key grounding point in this book. This orientation directly addresses the objective of health education cited by WHO (1974) as promoting in people a sense of individual and community responsibility for health, and an ability to participate in life constructively and purposefully.

PROGRAM DEVELOPMENT

Many distinctive approaches to health education planning are utilized, usually centering on many or all of the generic phases of assessing needs, stating the issues or problems to be addressed, developing goals and objectives, reviewing resources and barriers, determining methods, implementing, and evaluating. Specific examples include the PRECEDE approach (Green et al., 1980), emphasizing problem-aligned deductive diagnoses; the Ross and Mico (1980) model for health education planning which analyzes each planning phase through the dimensions of content (subject matter), method (steps and techniques), and process (interactions); and the Bates and Winder (1984) conceptual planning and resources development model which, in addition to the planning process, addresses five end results—health education plans, demonstration programs, operational programs, research programs, and information and statistics. Readers who have aligned themselves successfully with a particular health education planning process are advised to continue. Our focus in this book is to organize, describe, and demonstrate applications of structured needs assessment strategies which have had varying degrees of use in health education and health promotion throughout the past decade.

Tables 2.1-2.4 illustrate how needs assessment strategies fit into the bigger program planning picture, based upon insights offered by a national advisory committee assembled by the U.S. Health Resources Administration (1977). These tables present some basic program development considerations at each one of the planning stages. Though it may not be feasible for every programming effort to use all of the cited considerations at each stage, they do provide prompters for planning committee, and administrative discussions.

Table 2.1. *Program Development Considerations for Health Education and Health Promotion: Assessment.*

	Involvement	Defining Problems
Breadth	Representatives of key interests are involved in program development, especially those directly affected, and representatives from organizations likely to finance and implement programming. Planning committee is formed.	Key parts of the population are considered in defining the problems.
Scope	Consumer and provider inclusion in decision-making relates to the key phases of program development: defining problems, setting goals, designing plans, implementing plans, and evaluating programs.	Analyses are conducted to determine actual and projected gaps in (1) individual health-related behavior*, (2) health education practices and services, (3) health education resources, and (4) positive and negative forces affecting behavior, services, and resources.
Depth	Consumer and provider input for decision-making is received from those on the planning committee, as well as those external to the committee.	Valid, reliable and appropriate data and the opinions of key consumers and providers are ascertained.

*For example, promotion of vigorous well-being, prevention of disability and premature death, self-care of minor illnesses, appropriate use of services, carrying out of needed diagnostic and treatment procedures, and participation in community health program development.

Material adapted from the U. S. Health Resources Administration (DHEW) document, *Educating the Public About Health: A Planning Guide*, 1977.

The considerations listed under the "Defining Problems" column serve as a good introduction to some of the diverse issues related to needs assessments. Along with those cited, we would include the consideration that the reader recognize the various levels of needs one encounters when planning with others. Typically, when preparing to conduct a needs assessment, one focuses on the needs of a specified target audience. However, keep in mind that there are additional need considerations as one attempts to address program planning to its fullest extent; staff, volunteer, and organizational needs also need to be considered. A very high priority target audience need (as assessed by a health educator) may go unaddressed because colleagues have other commitments and interests, or because the need does not align well with agency priorities.

ADVISORY AND PLANNING COMMITTEES

One very helpful method to develop a clearer and more comprehensive planning approach is to establish a committee. Two types of committees can be formulated. An *advisory committee* usually is comprised of individuals who are in a position to periodically report on their actual experiences related to some common issue. Members of this committee

Table 2.2. *Program Development Considerations for Health Education and Health Promotion: Intervention Plan*

	Setting Goals and Objectives	Recommending Actions	Obtaining Resources
Scope	Priority decisions about goals and objectives are based on (1) gaps in health-related behavior*, and (2) weaknesses in the availability, accessibility, continuity, acceptability, quality**, and cost of health education and health promotion services.	Development of recommended actions is based on considering positive and negative forces affecting health-related behavior and health education services, alternative educational methods, possible supportive activities, gaps in resources, and needed advocacy.	Plans for resources are based on considering cost, personnel, organizational mechanisms, facilities, equipment, supplies, technical assistance, and legislation.
Appropriateness	Development of goals and objectives are based on relevance to people's values and desires, number of persons likely to benefit, amount of expected benefit per person in relation to cost, and byproducts that are expected to be more favorable than unfavorable.	Selection of recommended actions is based on relevance to people's desires, what is necessary and sufficient to achieve priority goals and objectives, the need to improve consumer participation in community health program development, consistency with knowledge about how people learn, more favorable than unfavorable byproducts, and the results of pretesting.	Selection of resources is based on relevance to people's desires, what is necessary and sufficient to carry out recommended actions, consideration of alternative types of resources, and consistency with knowledge about effective and efficient resource use.
Achievability	Goals and objectives are stated in terms of intended outcomes (not activities or processes). Desired changes are specific, and allow for quantitative measurement. Needed knowledge and resources are available. Affected population groups are indicated. Objectives include time targets.	Selection of recommended actions is based on the availability of knowledge and resources that show potential for their achievement. Progress is measurable. Affected population groups and expected impacts are indicated. Time targets are included.	

*For example, promotion of vigorous well-being, prevention of disability and premature death, self-care of minor illnesses, appropriate use of services, and carrying out of needed diagnostic and treatment procedures.

**Special consideration can be given here for the development of people's decision-making abilities.

Material adapted from the U. S. Health Resources Administration (DHEW) document, *Educating the Public About Health: A Planning Guide,* 1977.

Table 2.3. *Program Development Considerations for Health Education and Health Promotion: Implementation*

Planning for Implementation

Facilitation	The provider facilitates implementation of the plans through technical assistance, grants and contracts, taking public stands on relevant issues, requiring inclusion of high-quality health education components in proposals for use of federal funds and for new institutional services, helping coordinate health education activities, and advocating allocation of needed health education and health promotion resources by administrators, legislators, and others.
Commitment	Appropriate operating agencies make definite commitments for allocating needed resources to implement the plans.

Material adapted from the U. S. Health Resources Administration (DHEW) document, *Educating the Public About Health: A Planning Guide*, 1977.

Table 2.4. *Program Development Considerations for Health Education and Health Promotion: Evaluation*

Planning for Evaluation

Scope	Plans for evaluation of the programs call for assessing (1) achievement of objectives; (2) completion of actions and use of resources as planned; (3) relationships between achievement of objectives, carrying out of actions, and use of resources; (4) strengths and weaknesses of the program development processes; (5) favorable and unfavorable byproducts; and (6) the importance of this program as compared with others.
Appropriateness	Plans for evaluation of the programs (1) are relevant to the desires of the people being served, program funders, and program operators; (2) insure valid and reliable findings; (3) are expected to be worth the cost; and (4) are completed before the program is implemented.

Material adapted from the U. S. Health Resources Administration (DHEW) document, *Educating the Public About Health: A Planning Guide*, 1977.

are then able to offer their advice to a key individual who is bringing them together, or to another group which will be making programmatic decisions. This group is a *planning committee*, and can be made up of advisory committee members, experts, and agency staff. A planning committee may be episodic (with limited duration) or continuing (ongoing). There are instances where advisory committees are transformed into planning committees, with the addition of key people, so that a particular program can be developed. Both types of committees usually have one common denominator: they are task oriented. As pointed out by Trecker and Trecker (1979, p. 104), it usually will take a considerable amount of time, planning, and thinking to develop the right committee structure and recruit those who will serve. These authors offer a helpful citation of steps to be taken for committee formation within the context of the community change process (Trecker and Trecker, 1979, pp. 104-118; 148-207).

Both types of committees are important to longterm needs assessment processes. They enable firsthand insights and experiences to be offered; they encourage brainstorming; and, particularly in the planning committee process, there can be an early commitment by committee members to undertake key program planning responsibilities at appropriate times. However, working with a committee can be a two-edged sword. As Poole and Hirokawa (1986) have stated:

"the unique chemistry of social interaction can distill the best that each member has to offer, creating a resonance of ideas and a synthesis of viewpoints. A different chemistry can stop the reaction and contaminate the product with erratic reasoning or low commitment." (p. 15)

They continue, citing the value of understanding both the strategic (task oriented) and symbolic forms of communication taking place in groups.

One can find many examples of advisory and planning groups which have a needs assessment responsibility. British patient participation groups have been officially encouraged and instituted as neighborhood-based advisory committees which meet regularly to identify local health care related needs (Richardson and Bray, 1987). In 1978, a National Association for Patient Participation was established in Great Britain to provide a link between already existing patient participation groups and to foster new ones. Along with the solicitation of the patient's opinions regarding the quality of health care experienced, these groups also provide avenues for health education programming, and the provision of voluntary services to other patients (for example, transportation to the hospital). As another example, the City of Winnipeg in 1972 established Resident Advisory Groups as a part of their already-instituted community committees (aligned with city wards) in order to receive continuing insights into neighborhood needs (Axworthy et al., 1973). Needs were then reported based upon the uniquely different neighborhood experiences of distinctive environments, ethnic mixtures, socioeconomic mixtures, and political compositions.

PRELIMINARY OBSERVATIONS

As health professionals we gain insights from a variety of sources. In Chapter 1 we referred to insights derived from experience and intuition—understandings which have arisen through our collective professional involvement in health-related matters, rather than as specific results of pre-planned needs assessments. These insights are important in our work, and form somewhat of a backdrop against which we can play the findings of our intentional needs assessment efforts. In a more structured fashion, additional background and supplemental information can be garnered through a review of *secondary information,* which offers social and health indicators for inferential purposes.

Important insights can be derived from analyzing raw data and published data summaries. These are termed secondary information sources since the analyst did not collect and compile the original data. Sources of these data compilations include libraries, reports of experts and authorities, agency and organizational reports, and commercial information services (Stewart, 1984). Compiled health-related information abounds, as exemplified by the U.S. Census Reports, *Morbidity and Mortality Weekly Reports* (MMWR) from the Centers for Disease Control (CDC), and the *Monthly Vital Statistics Report* (MVSR) from the National Center for Health Statistics (NCHS) at the CDC. The importance of reviewing the data provided by the NCHS was heralded by the editor of *American Journal of Public Health* in stating that the "output of NCHS forms the very core of public health . . ." as that journal inaugurated in December 1987, a continuing new section entitled "New from NCHS" (Yankauer, 1987).

Secondary information can be derived from local, state, national, and international sources. This information can be directly obtained from the publisher (in many instances free of charge and in an ongoing manner from public agencies) or indirectly through a library. In some instances, specific documents will be on hand or easily obtainable. However, in other circumstances, one will have a general idea about the type of information which is required, but will not be able to cite a specific reference. In these cases, guides and directories are most beneficial. At the national level, examples of helpful guides would be the *Guide to Federal Statistics, A Selected List,* published by the Bureau of the U.S. Census, and the *Guide to U.S. Government Statistics.* A useful international document is the *Directory of United Nations Information Systems and Services.*

Examples of data sources at the local level include those maintained by a vital statistics section of a local health department (and usually reported in an annual report), and regional data collected by a Health Systems Agency (HSA). It is important to note that HSA's have commissioned regional needs assessments which collect data above and beyond vital statistics. It is advised to determine if there is an operational HSA in your region, and then investigate the data which has been collected. At the national level, valuable data and informational updates are provided by the previously-described MMWR, MVSR, and NCHS Reports. Additional resources include the *Statistical Abstract of the United States* and special reports incorporating data from Standard Metropolitan Statistical Areas (SMSA's), with each SMSA being a single county or cluster of contiguous counties which has at least one city with a minimum of 50,000 people. Specific international resources highly regarded are those provided by the World Health Organization (WHO), such as *World Health Statistics* and the *Weekly Epidemiological Record*.

These types of data provide health-related statistical information. Additionally, one can examine demographic data which provide information on population patterns, absenteeism records for work and school, income distribution, and political preferences. When we examine this broader context of statistical and demographic data "that identify the size and characteristics of population groups with particular needs, the symptoms of those needs, and the scope of the problem" as Witkin (1984, p. 100) has stated, we are addressing social indicators. Witkin (1984) also clarifies that there is a distinction between indicators and indices, where the former are data that have been selected, corrected, and refined, and the latter are composed of combinations of two or more indicators. Social indicators can be subjective or objective data, direct or indirect measures, and descriptive (descriptions about social characteristics) or analytic (relationships among characteristics). Overall, examination of social indicators can provide the health professional with an understanding of the community context in which he or she is working. Questions may arise which will then lead to potential clarification through the structured needs assessment strategies. Social indicators also may support and supplement the results derived from the structured strategies.

KEY INFORMANT INSIGHTS

Another process for gaining preliminary information and insights is through contact with selected individuals who are able to express their perceptions of the needs of others. These individuals, termed key informants, include community leaders, health and human service professionals, leaders of religious organizations, public officials, educators, and the like. One's planning or advisory committee can be approached to develop a list of possible candidates, with the eventual selection based upon established criteria, such as: (1) whether the person's views or actions influence others, (2) the level of knowledge of the community, (3) the degree to which the person represents a particular group, (4) the level of knowledge about the service agency, and (5) a person's residence ("How to Use the Key Informant Survey Technique," 1985).

When identified, these individuals are usually contacted through one of the interview or survey strategies detailed in the subsequent chapters. Williams (1978, p. 93) has cautioned that while this approach can provide a comprehensive and manageable assessment of the need perceptions for consumers, high-risk groups, professionals, and others, if it is used in isolation, it has the potential for generalizations, influence of vested interests, and avoidance of those actually experiencing problems. Thus, when possible, one should consider the key informant information as a starting point which is to be followed with more direct assessments of the target audience.

NEEDS PRIORITIZATION

Once data are collected through the secondary sources and/or through the structured strategies (to be detailed in forthcoming chapters), analyses of the meaning of the data must take place. It is strongly recommended that these procedures be established prior to the collection of the data, as part of the overall needs assessment plan. Additionally, one must keep in mind that initially the prioritization should be based upon the needs of the target group, as distinguished from those of the service providers. In each of the subsequent chapters, we address specific analytic procedures through the sections entitled, "Using the Results."

The simplest method of prioritizing is to have the assessed needs ranked by target group members and representatives. Using this process, individuals are asked to rank the top five needs (or some other predetermined number) out of all of those presented. In analyzing the group results, each need has the potential of receiving a series of rankings which can then be averaged for a mean rank, or weighted (e.g., in a 1-5 scale, a rank of 1 will have a weighting of 5; a rank of 2 will have a weighting of 4, and so forth; the weights are then added together for each need, with the highest-valued need being top-ranked). If it is deemed advisable to have several target group clusters of members and representatives rank the same list of assessed needs (typically because of the complexity of the issues and/or settings), one could very well end up with several different ranking patterns. An example of this was presented by Kimmel (1977) in which three groups in Florida (clients, community members, and key informants) were asked to rank the top five priority needs. The results showed that the clients and community members had concurrence on what four of the five were, but they were not ranked in the same order (i.e., 1,769 clients ranked the top five in priority order as routine dental care, financial assistance, food stamps, utility problems, and transportation; 1,187 community members rank ordered the needs as routine dental care, food stamps, financial assistance, information and referral, and transportation). The third group, key informants, had cited unemployment, child abuse, malnutrition, transportation, and low-income medical care, in rank order. How would one make a decision based upon these data? Typically, if the data are evolving from different samples of the same type of group, need statements can be combined mathematically and general need areas formulated (see Chapter 6). This then enables the decision-maker to review the final rankings from all of the collected data. However, the above example shows data coming from three distinctive groups, usually necessitating more complex analytic procedures.

Due to the complexity of needs which can be assessed through various strategies, no one analytic process can serve all purposes. Thus, for more in-depth discussions regarding selected procedures, the reader may wish to review Dever (1984, pp. 65-66, 117-131), McKillip (1987, pp. 105-119), and Witkin (1984, pp. 206-240). A helpful model developed by Sork (1982) at the University of British Columbia is reviewed by Witkin (1984, pp. 230-232). The model offers a systematic process for determining priorities with a certain degree of built-in flexibility. The basic steps include the following:

1. Select Appropriate Criteria. The two general categories of importance and feasibility are suggested, with examples of the former being number of people affected, magnitude of the difference between present and future status, and alignment with organizational goals; examples of the latter being efficacy level of health educational and promotional intervention, resource availability, and perceived ability to change.

2. Assign Relative Importance to Each Criterion. Criteria are weighted equally or by degree on a scale of 1 to 10, with the criterion of least weight (1) identified first, and then each subsequent criterion compared against it, so that the criterion weighted 10 is ten times the weight of 1.

3. Apply Each Criterion to Each Need. A separate list of priorities is established for each criterion used, with priority values expressed numerically or through descriptors such as high, medium, and low.

4. Combine Individual Values to yield a Total Priority Value for Each Need. One approach here is to add weighted ranks and establish mean ranks for each identified need.

5. Arrange Needs for Highest to Lowest Total Priority Value and

Indicate How Priorities Will be Used. Resource alignment with the identified needs can be established in this step.

From another vantage point, some decision-makers may wish to review the assessed needs in a highly qualitative fashion. Using this approach, special criteria can be established as questions against which the needs will be reviewed through group discussion. Examples of such questions are offered in a manual offered by the Ministry of Education in Victoria, British Columbia (Lund and McGechaen, 1981, pp. 16-17) and reviewed by Witkin (1984, p. 230):

- Does the target group recognize this need?
- How many people are affected?
- What would be the consequences if this need is not met?
- Is this a need that can be met by an educational activity?
- Does this need coincide with your department or institution's program policies? If not, what are the reasons for the present policies? What procedures are available for influencing needed change?
- Can you rely on co-sponsorship or cooperation with another agency?
- Is this a critical need that should be met before other educational needs are addressed?
- Will resources (funds, staff) be adequate to meet those needs?

Using this approach, health professionals have the opportunity to discuss multiple responses to the questions, as well as the various rationales for those responses. While this approach typically takes more time, the complexity of the issues being addressed could well merit it.

SUMMARY

The context of a health professional's program planning experiences, observations, and secondary information sources provides a valuable framework for active involvement in health education and health promotion. This context also enables the professional to make decisions about more appropriate next steps for structured needs assessment strategies. Chapters 3 through 10 will detail these strategies by addressing selection considerations, along with preparation and implementation procedures. Table 2.5 delineates the manner in which the structured strategies will be addressed.

Table 2.5. *Structured Needs Assessment Strategies for Health Education and Health Promotion*

Process Category	Types
Assessments with Individuals	—Single-Step Surveys (Chapter 3) —Multi-Step Survey-Delphi (Chapter 4) —Interviewing (Chapter 5)
Assessments with Groups	—Nominal Group Process (Chapter 6) —Focus Group Process (Chapter 7) —Other Group Assessment Processes (Chapter 8)
Self-Directed Assessments	—Inventories (Chapter 9) —Observational Methods (Chapter 10)

Part II

Assessments with Individuals

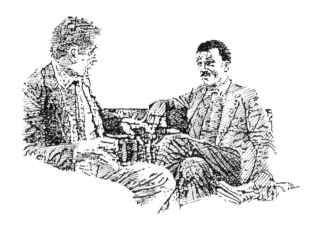

The three chapters in Part II address the needs assessments the health professional can conduct with individuals. This approach is accomplished through surveys and interviewing. Many surveys and interviews involve just one contact with the participants; we also will describe the Delphi survey strategy which involves several contacts with the same participants, on an individual basis. After reviewing each strategy, we will offer suggestions for preparing and conducting needs assessment, and using the results.

3

Single-Step Surveys

INTRODUCTION

Surveys are one of the oldest methods for gathering information. Face-to-face surveys date back to the ancient world. The Bible records a census of the Israelites. The Roman Empire was conducting a census when Christ was born. Skipping a few centuries, perhaps the first mail survey was King Philip II of Spain's census of New World possessions, conducted by official courier in 1577 (Erdos, 1983, pp. 1-2). Telephone surveys are a more recent phenomenon. One of the first, and perhaps the most infamous, phone survey was conducted by the *Literary Digest* in 1936. That survey predicted a landslide victory in the Presidential election for Alf Landon over Franklin Roosevelt (Frey, 1983, pp. 18-19).

Surveys have changed since these early examples. Today they are widely used—mail surveys, telephone surveys, and face-to-face surveys. For some time following the *Literary Digest* survey, telephone surveys were considered less reliable than mail surveys. Since not all homes had phones, telephone surveys tended to include primarily educated and at least middle income people. As a result, surveys requiring a more representative cross section of the population would be invalid. Face-to-face surveys were preferred, since better coverage of the population could be obtained. Mail surveys also were shown to achieve better results than phone surveys (Frey, 1983, p. 19).

Phone surveys, however, have improved their ability to collect reliable and valid information. The telephone has become a standard in American households. The 1980 United States Census showed that 98% of the households had a telephone, compared to 36% in 1936. Although unlisted numbers are increasing, random digit dialing and other related techniques enable surveyors to reach people who opt out of directory listings.

Surveys have been widely used to assess educational needs. Mail surveying is probably the most frequently-used strategy. Keep in mind that surveys are something you can easily do. You do not have to be an expert researcher to conduct a good survey. You can follow the steps outlined in this chapter and get good results.

REVIEWING AND SELECTING A STRATEGY
Mail Survey
Advantages
Low cost. All surveys have similar basic costs, which include developing and producing the questionnaire, analyzing the data, and communicating the results. Where they differ primarily is in collecting data. A mail survey costs the least to collect data. The only direct cost is postage for mailings. As a result, less personnel are needed. For many needs assessments, one person with a few basic research skills can conduct the entire survey from start to finish. Larger projects may require assistance from staff members with expertise in questionnaire design and data analysis. Yet the entire project can be accomplished from one central office.

Wide distribution. To reach a diverse group of people, a mail survey is best. Some people may not have a telephone, but they do receive mail delivery if they have an address. Gaining access to people through face-to-face surveys is becoming more difficult, as discussed below.

Valid information. A mail survey provides the best chance of getting a truthful answer, especially when asking potentially threatening questions. The respondents can offer their answers in the privacy of their homes or workplaces. They do not have to muster the courage to respond to an interviewer.

A mail survey also provides a better opportunity for a thoughtful reply. Respondents can complete the survey when they have the time and perspective to give the best answer, rather than responding on-the-spot to an interviewer's questions. Also, a mail survey eliminates the bias and influence that an interviewer brings to a telephone or face-to-face situation.

Disadvantages
Lengthy process. Although a mail questionnaire saves money and personnel, you lose time waiting for the surveys to be returned. To obtain a good response, a mail survey typically takes three or four months to complete (Frey, 1983, p. 33). Of that time, two months or more is spent waiting for the returns from your initial mailing and one or two follow-up mailings.

Lower response rate. A mail survey generally will attract fewer respondents than a telephone or face-to-face survey. In fact, the response rate is declining for the general public, because of increasing concerns about privacy, and perhaps because of overuse (Frey, 1983, p. 39). A 50% response rate is considered very good (Erdos, 1983, p. 4). Higher responses of 60% to 75% are possible (Erdos, 1983, p. 4; Dillman, 1978, p. 51), especially when surveying a relatively homogeneous group and using thorough follow-up techniques.

Number and type of questions limited. Generally, the shorter the survey and the simpler the questions, the better the response. Respondents will take more time for a phone or face-to-face survey than they will for a mail survey. For the general public, your questionnaire should be no more than four pages. For a relatively homogeneous group, however, a 12-page survey is not out of the question (Frey, 1983, pp. 48-49; Sudman and Bradburn, 1983, p. 227). Only a few open-ended questions should be used, since too many will discourage responses. Complex questions are difficult to include, because you cannot ask follow-up questions to clarify the meaning of responses.

No control over answers. You cannot control who answers your questionnaire. You may send it to a household with explicit instructions for a teenager to complete, but you do not know whether she completed the questionnaire or her father did. You cannot keep a respondent from consulting with another person before giving an answer, nor can you encourage a respondent to answer a question instead of skipping it.

Mailing list required. Although a mail survey can reach a diverse group of people, complete mailing lists are not always readily available. If they are available, they may not be accurate (Frey, 1983, p. 37). The more accurate ones may be expensive to obtain. What seemed to be an inexpensive survey may become costly.

Telephone survey

Advantages

Shorter process. The preparation time for a telephone survey can be slightly longer than for a mail survey, but data collection is more direct and controllable. You can call the participants and have the information immediately, rather than having extended and sporadic mail responses.

Better response rate. Answering questions over the phone takes less effort than sitting down to complete a questionnaire. As long as you contact people at a convenient time, you can expect greater participation in a phone survey than in a mail survey. Response rates as high as 80% to 85% are possible (Dillman, 1978, p. 51), especially when calling individuals who identify with the project or have some stake in its outcome. Response rates from the general public may be lower.

More and different questions possible. Participants typically are willing to answer more questions for a phone survey than for a mail survey. For the general public, a survey lasting 10 to 20 minutes is reasonable. For relatively homogeneous groups, telephone surveys have lasted as long as 50 minutes to an hour, with good results. Participants will tolerate open-ended questions much better than for a mail survey. Complex questions are easier to ask, since follow-up questions are possible.

Better control over answers. Unlike mail questionnaires, which are out of one's control when mailed, the telephone offers an opportunity to verify an appropriate respondent. The telephone process also can discourage consultation with others and encourage responses to all questions.

Good access to respondents. Although one can reach fewer people by phone than by mail, a very high percentage of American households have access to a telephone. Special dialing techniques described later in this chapter, can be used to reach people with unlisted numbers.

Disadvantages

More costly. Collecting data typically is more expensive than for a mail survey. If long distance calls are necessary, the cost will be much more than postage to mail a questionnaire. One person may be able to do all the interviews, but extra help is often needed. Conducting interviews is much more time consuming than tracking mail questionnaires. The extra interviewers may need to be paid for their training and interviewing time. For a large project involving several interviewers, additional supervisory help will be required.

Less valid information. If you ask potentially threatening questions, one stands a better chance of receiving a socially desirable response by phone than by mail. Participants find threatening questions more difficult to answer candidly when talking to an interviewer (Frey, 1983, p. 54; Sudman and Bradburn, 1983, pp. 277-278).

Face-to-face Survey

Advantages

Best opportunity for questioning. A face-to-face survey is the best way to administer a lengthy questionnaire. Although a half hour limit is desirable (Sudman and Bradburn, 1983, p. 227), face-to-face surveys lasting an hour or more are not uncommon (Frey, 1983, p. 48). Open-ended and complex questions are best handled in a face-to-face survey, since follow-up questions are easily asked.

Most control over answers. Compared to a telephone survey, there is more assurance that the appropriate person is answering the questions and not consulting with other people. Using both verbal and non-verbal expression, one also can offer greater encouragement to answer all questions.

Disadvantages

Most costly. Since interviewers must travel, often from house to house, to collect data, travel time and expenses can be significant. The interview itself tends to take longer in person than over the phone. Although one person can conduct an entire mail or telephone survey, a face-to-face survey will require at least one other person to assist with interviews. Large projects require several interviewers, as well as supervisory help. Training is more extensive, since interviewers must make judgments in the field without the benefit of consulting with a supervisor.

Least valid information. A face-to-face survey is the most difficult setting for asking potentially threatening questions. Participants are most tempted to give a socially desirable answer when they have to face another person (Frey, 1983, p. 54; Sudman and Bradburn, 1983, pp. 277-278).

Becoming difficult to gain access to participants. Historically, face-to-face surveys have offered good access to the public. They do not require a good mailing list or telephone directory. Interviewers can go directly to the people; they can ring doorbells or solicit participation at shopping centers. Over the years, they have yielded the highest response rate (Frey, 1983, p. 39; Dillman, 1978, p. 51).

More recently, face-to-face surveys have become difficult to conduct. Some people are concerned about privacy and security. More women have entered the workforce, leaving fewer people available at home during the day. Evenings are possible, but families often have evening activities. Interviewers are reluctant to venture into some neighborhoods in metropolitan areas. Public places also are difficult for conducting a survey, because people are often in a hurry.

When considering the advantages and disadvantages of mail, phone, and face-to-face surveys, five criteria need to be kept in mind: the type of information needed, from whom it will be collected, the money you have available, the time available, and the personnel who can assist you.

1. Type of information

    If the information you need is potentially threatening to the participants, especially information on behavior patterns, a mail survey should yield the most valid data. If you need to ask complex questions which require follow-up questions for clarification, a face-to-face survey offers the best situation. Open-ended questions also are best handled face-to-face. If your survey is lengthy, a face-to-face survey is best, followed by a telephone survey.

2. Audience

    If you plan to survey the general public, a telephone survey or face-to-face survey typically yields a higher response than a mail survey. If you plan to survey low literate people or those not skilled in the use of English, a face-to-face survey is best. These individuals may not be able to complete a mail survey and may not feel comfortable talking to a stranger on the phone. For a professional audience, however, a telephone survey may be best. Professional people are used to giving information over the phone.

3. Money

   If money is in short supply, a mail survey may be your only option. A simple telephone survey, however, can be inexpensive, as long as too many long distance calls are not required.

4. Time

   If you need to do the survey quickly, use the telephone. You will need time, however, to recruit and train interviewers.

5. Personnel

   A mail survey requires the least personnel, while the face-to-face survey requires the most. A face-to-face survey also requires the most qualified interviewers, since they are on their own when conducting the survey.

Finally, keep two other important considerations in mind, regardless which survey method one uses to assess needs. Remember that people respond based on how they feel at the time of the survey. They will not necessarily do something about their needs at a later time. Also, remember that surveys have been widely used to assess educational needs. What once was a novelty may now be overused.

PREPARING FOR THE ASSESSMENT

The preparation phase is similar for mail, telephone, and face-to-face surveys. We will discuss the general steps; for some steps, we will suggest considerations which apply to a particular survey method.

Decide What You Want to Know

It is important to clearly identify what you need to learn from the individuals you plan to survey. Having a clear idea before beginning can save valuable time for all concerned.

Decide whether you need to ask people what they know or what their attitudes are about a certain subject, or for them to describe certain behaviors. If you plan to ask about behavior, consider whether describing this behavior will be threatening to the individual.

Develop a Budget

Before you begin developing the survey, find out how much financial support is available. You have an approximate budget in mind, which helped you select which survey method to use. Now put the budget in final form, including personnel costs for collecting and analyzing data, printing the questionnaire and final report, postage, long distance telephone calls, travel expenses, and computer analysis. Having a thorough budget will help you decide, for example, how many people to employ, how many people to survey, and how much data analysis to do.

Prepare your Questions

Before rushing ahead to develop your own questions, consider whether someone else has developed questions you could use. For a needs assessment, existing questions may be difficult to find which fit your situation exactly. They may be modified, however, to fit your project. Or they can suggest other questions you might develop yourself. (Review Chapter 2 for possible sources, particularly the secondary references.)

When developing questions, keep in mind the type of survey which will be used, who will be surveyed, and how the collected data will be analyzed. Remember that a mail survey should include primarily closed questions, which give the respondent a choice of answers to select (true or false, multiple choice, or rank ordering several possibilities or situations). Open-ended questions require participants to generate answers. For a mail survey, limit the number of open-ended questions. The shorter the answer required, the better. By contrast, telephone and face-to-face surveys can handle more less-focused, open-ended questions.

The people you survey also affect the type of questions you plan to develop. If you plan to survey a sample of the general public, remember that many of them will not be highly motivated to participate. They will respond best to closed questions. Also, they may refuse to answer threatening questions about their behavior. If you plan to survey people who are highly-motivated to participate, either because they identify with your efforts or have a stake in how the information will be used, open-ended questions are more appropriate. These people will take more time to respond in a thoughtful manner.

How you plan to analyze your data also should influence the questions you develop. Open-ended questions may yield excellent information, but they take much more time and skill to analyze. If you are short on time, money, or skilled personnel, you may need to limit the number of open-ended questions.

Test and Modify Your Questions

After spending time and energy developing questions, you may have very good questions. However, they need to be submitted to careful scrutiny to become even better. At this stage, other people can spot ambiguities or suggest alternate wording to clarify and improve the questions. When developing your questions, share them with as many colleagues as you can. Include those people who will analyze the data. Ask them to critique the questions and suggest ways to improve the wording, and ask them to tell you what they think the questions mean. Try not to worry about criticism of your questions. Think of them as first efforts, rather than finished masterpieces.

Develop a Draft of Your Survey

Keep your respondents in mind as you develop your questionnaire. You want to ensure their participation from start to finish. Begin with questions that are relatively easy to answer. Like a long distance runner, the respondent needs to warm up and get into the flow of the survey. Use closed questions at this early stage.

Place difficult or potentially threatening questions near the middle of the survey. Open-ended questions also work best in the middle. You want the respondents to answer these questions after they are warmed up, but before they become tired. Ask demographic questions at the end of the survey. Questions about the respondent's age, income, and family status, also can be threatening. Demographic questions also can be answered quickly. When completion is in sight, having just a few quick questions left can help.

When reviewing the questions, continually ask yourself why. Ask yourself why you need the answer to each question. More importantly, ask yourself what you will do with the answer to each question. If you have no specific use for the answer, or you are unsure, omit the question. This will save time and effort for your participants, and you. The more data collected, the more data to summarize and analyze. You only have so much time and money to devote to this project; use them wisely. Aim to have a few good questions.

Pilot Test Your Survey

For an extensive research project, rigorous pilot-testing is strongly recommended. Sudman and Bradburn (1983, p. 282) recommend several different steps. Included are peer critique of a draft questionnaire, revision and testing on friends and colleagues, pilot testing on a small sample of respondents, written comments from surveyors and respondents, and further pilot testing.

If you cannot afford extensive pilot testing, try to find a small group of people to practice taking your survey. Try to simulate the conditions under which the final draft will be administered. Select a small sample of people, typically no more than 20, who are similar to those who will complete the final version. Administer the survey, using the same directions you will use later. Include an extra page at the end for them to comment about the questionnaire. Have them identify confusing questions and state the reasoning they used to answer them. Also, ask them to critique certain questions and suggest any improvements.

Once you have completed the pilot surveys, analyze the data just as you would the final version. Determine whether the questions are giving the information you need, and if any rewriting is necessary.

Develop Coding and Data Analysis Procedures

Before designing the final survey, think through how you will analyze the data. Plan for statistical analysis, if appropriate. Consult with the staff who will handle the data analysis. They can suggest the best way to form the survey to make the data as easy to understand and categorize as possible.

Another important reason for planning the data analysis procedures at this stage is to ensure that it is done promptly. You could become very involved in collecting data, and the data could sit on the shelf too long before being used. *Plan* your entire approach and analysis.

Design the Final Survey

Consider three groups of people when designing the final questionnaire: the respondents, the interviewer (if used), and the data processors.

For a mail survey, give the respondents primary consideration. Remember that length can be a problem, especially for the general public. Design your survey to look as professional as possible. If the budget allows, printing the questionnaire in booklet form may get the best response. When designing the questionnaire, the objective is to obtain the best response for the money available. A 7 x 10 inch booklet format has been found to get a good response. If that is not realistic, an 8 ½ x 11 inch size is acceptable. Surveys larger than that have been shown to get lower responses. A neutral color (tan, ivory, or grey) also may enhance the response (Erdos, 1983, pp. 39-40).

The most important consideration, however, is that your survey is easy to read. Use a relatively large and readable typeface. Do not try to shorten the survey be reducing the type. What you gain by having fewer pages, you will lose by having difficult type to read. A slightly longer survey is better than type that is too small. Also, be sure you include clear directions. If respondents must skip certain questions based on how other questions are answered, make sure these directions are clearly and boldly identified.

For telephone and face-to-face surveys, give the interviewers primary consideration. A good design can help alleviate some of the pressure, which is a normal part of conducting a survey. Length of the questionnaire is no longer as important. Instead, make sure you include clear directions for the interviewers and enough space to record answers. Design the booklet to be easy to use during the survey. Use extra white space to set the questions apart from each other.

Design all surveys to enhance good data analysis. Place the answers in a consistent location, so they can be picked up easily. If the survey will be computer scored, include the appropriate field numbers. Readers desiring additional detail for survey design procedures are referred to more in-depth discussions by Dever (1980, pp. 147-168) and Abramson (1979, pp. 99-190).

CONDUCTING THE ASSESSMENT

Although the preparation phase is similar for mail, telephone, and face-to-face surveys, the conducting phase varies significantly.

Mail Survey

Select a sample of respondents. Unless you have already designated a group to survey, you will have to select a sample from a large population. Decide how many respondents you want to survey. (Make sure your budget can handle the numbers.) Then, select a sample. Usually, a systematic sample is drawn by selecting names from a mailing list (Frey, 1983, p. 65).

First, determine the size of the list and the size of the sample needed. Divide the list size by the sample size to determine the size of the interval between the names to be selected. Pick a number at random between one and the size of the interval, inclusive. Select this number from a table of random numbers. This number is the number of the first name selected from your mailing list. Then skip as many names as the size of the interval and select that name. Proceed through the entire list to complete your sample, selecting names at each interval. For example, if you want to select 50 participants from a mailing list of 500 people, the interval size is 10. Randomly select a number between one and 10, inclusive. If that number is seven, choose the seventh person on the list. Then choose the 17th person, the 27th person, and so on through the entire list, until you have selected 50 people. For additional sampling procedures, see Green and Lewis (1982, pp. 223-240).

Mail the questionnaires. Include a brief cover letter which explains who is conducting the survey, why it is important, and the benefits that will result. Explain how the respondents were selected, and assure them their responses will be kept confidential. Before sending the questionnaires, code them inconspicuously with a number so you can tell who has and has not responded. Assure the respondents that this number is for coding purposes only.

Indicate a date by which the respondents should return the questionnaire. Two or three weeks is a good length of time. Busier people may not be able to complete the survey immediately, but you do not want the questionnaire forgotten. Include a stamped, self-addressed envelope for return of the survey.

Send a follow-up mailing. Most of the surveys returned after a first mailing will arrive within three weeks (Erdos, 1983, p. 131). Log in the returns by code number. Three or four weeks after the first mailing, send a reminder letter to those who have not responded with another coded copy of the questionnaire. A simpler follow-up approach is to send a reminder postcard to everyone, noting to those who have already responded to disregard the notice.

Telephone Survey

Select a sample of respondents. If you plan to survey employees or members of an organization, you first will need to obtain its staff directory or membership list. Then, draw a systematic sample from this population.

If you plan to survey the general public, the community telephone directory is the most obvious source of phone numbers. This directory, however, will not include unlisted numbers. Several techniques exist for gaining access to unlisted numbers, but a simple and effective method is adding a digit (Frey, 1983, pp. 67-77). Draw a systematic sample of telephone numbers, and then add one digit to every number. That way you are not limited to phone numbers in the directory.

Select and train the interviewers. Explain the purpose of the survey, who is conducting it, why it is important, and the resulting benefits. Give the interviewers written instructions on how to conduct the surveys. Include how many attempts to make to reach a participant before proceeding to another, how to introduce the survey, how to handle ambiguous answers, and how to record the data. Have the interviewers practice and critique one another. If possible, have them practice by telephone on people who are similar to participants in the survey.

Collect and record the data. The interviewers should proceed through the survey, following the directions on the questionnaire and the instructions they received during training. If possible, have all interviewers place calls from a central location during the same period of time. That way one supervisor can be present to handle any problems that arise.

Face-to-Face Survey

Decide who and where to survey. A variety of possibilities exist for conducting a face-to-face survey. You can select a systematic sample of participants from a mailing list or telephone directory and then arrange to survey in person. Or, you can interview the oldest female member of every fifth household in a neighborhood, or you can randomly select people at a shopping mall or on a street corner.

Select and train interviewers. The selection of interviewers is most critical for a face-to-face survey. The interviewers need to enjoy and feel comfortable in a face-to-face situation. Since they will conduct these surveys with little or no supervision, they need the ability to exercise good judgment. Once the interviewers are selected, the training is similar to phone survey training.

Collect and record the data. Give the interviewers explicit instructions on who and where to survey. The data collection is similar to the telephone survey.

USING THE RESULTS

Feeling tired after a sustained preparation and data collection effort, you may prefer to put the data inside while you catch up with other projects. However, it is important to maintain the momentum you have established. If you set the data aside now, you may find it difficult to get back to the project later. Having planned your data analysis earlier will help you keep going now and work through any slump that might occur.

Most data you collect from a survey will be quantitative data. You will need some way to summarize these numbers for your planning committee or other interested groups. Sophisticated statistical tests typically are not necessary for needs assessment. As discussed in Chapter 1, needs assessment is not the same as rigorous academic research. Although some of the same research skills are used, the data are used differently.

Simple descriptive statistics are usually sufficient for a needs assessment. Perform the following calculations.

1. Tabulate frequency distributions.
   Count the number of times each response occurs for each item. For a small survey, count these responses manually. For a large survey, use a computer to enter the data and summarize frequencies.
2. Determine the range of responses.
   Note the lowest response and the highest response for each item.
3. Calculate the most appropriate measure of central tendency.
   The mean is most typically used. It is most appropriate when you have a relatively narrow range of responses with a relatively even distribution. The mean is simply the arithmetic average of all responses to the item. To calculate the mean, add the scores and divide by the number of responses.

Sometimes the median and the mode are more helpful statistics than the mean. The median is most simply understood as the middle score in the distribution. It is a more appropriate measure of central tendency when some scores are skewed much higher or much lower than the rest of the scores. To determine the median, arrange all responses in ascending order from low to high. Count the scores, beginning with the lowest score, until you reach the middle score. That is the median. If you have an even number of scores, determine the point halfway between the two middle scores.

The mode is the response that occurs most frequently. It is an appropriate measure of central tendency when one particular response to an item is clearly more frequent than any other. Using the mean or median in this case may not show the importance of this response.

Although most survey data are quantitative, some data may be qualitative (words to analyze, instead of numbers). If you have surveyed only a few people, you can handle open-ended questions with verbal responses by simply listing verbatim the responses received. Typically the open-ended questions from a survey will be focused, such that responses will be relatively short and to the point.

Another way to handle verbal responses, especially when you have a large number of participants, is to combine similar responses. You then will have more of a summary statement. Indicate how many people offered this kind of a response. If you do summarize responses, be careful not to collapse similar statements too much. You can lose some of the meaning. The more you summarize, the more you introduce your own interpretation into the responses. You want to present the responses as faithfully as possible in the way they were received. Later, you can add your own interpretation.

If you have a wide variation of responses to a particular question, you may need to do more combining and interpreting. First, read quickly through all responses to the item to get a feel for the range of responses. As you read, think of possible categories and jot them down. Then develop an initial list categories. Reread the responses and count the number of responses that fit each category. As you make this first attempt at categorizing the responses, you may think of additional categories that fit the data better. Add these categories to your list, rather than forcing a response into a category which seems to distort the meaning. After you have completed this second reading of the data, you may want to combine similar categories or rearrange them in some way. Finally, some miscellaneous responses may not fit any category. Report these responses separately. After this qualitative analysis, you may want to report the results in some quantitative form. Use frequency tabulations, range, and measures of central tendency.

The final step in this phase is to share the results with your planning committee or other interested groups. Remember, we cautioned earlier against collecting too much data. If you collected too much data, it will

Figure 3.1. *Needs Assessment Survey Example.*

COMMUNITY HEALTH EDUCATION NEEDS ASSESSMENT

Please review each of the topics listed below. Choose the five topics of most interest to you. You will note that you can add your own topic in the last space if you wish. Rank the five topics accordingly:

1 = highest need/interest
5 = lowest need/interest

A. Options in Elder Care: Where Are Your Aging Parents Going to Live? _____

B. Stresses and Strengths of Multi-generational Families _____

C. Success Oriented Gerontology: Expanding Our Knowledge of Healthy Old Age _____

D. Wellness and Spirituality _____

E. Examining Spirituality: Beyond Traditional Religions _____

F. Positive Self Concept and Self-Esteem: The Greatest Gift Parents Can Give Their Children _____

G. Learning to Like Yourself: Self Concept Improvement in Adults _____

H. Promoting Your Employees Mental Health (For Supervisors, Managers, etc.) _____

I. Ethical Issues in Death and Dying: Removal of Life Support, Organ Donation, Living Wills, etc. _____

J. Women/Men. Changing Roles, Relationships and Expectations _____

K. Playfulness, Humor and Healthy Lifestyles: How to Get Some Laughter Back Into Your Life _____

L. Eating Disorders: Helping Parents Recognize Early Symptoms _____

M. Human Sexuality: Couples Enduring and Endearing _____

N. Examining Your Health Potential: How to Expand on Your Healthy Behaviors (a wellness appraisal tool to be used) _____

O. Prevention of Teenage Suicide _____

P. Other: _____

Please indicate here if you would be interested in planning, hosting or co-sponsoring one of the above workshops.

Yes_____   TOPIC _____

Your Name and Phone No. _____

Used with permission of D. Kerns, Community Health, University of Wisconsin-La Crosse Extended Education and University of Wisconsin-Extension.

Figure 3.2. *Needs Assessment Survey Results.*

A) 1 – 7
   2 – 4
   3 – 3
   4 – 2
   5 – 2

I) 1 – 5
   2 – 5
   3 – 4
   4 – 7
   5 – 3

B) 1 – 3
   2 – 5
   3 – 3
   4 – 1
   5 – 5

J) 1 – 7
   2 – 8
   3 – 6
   4 – 6
   5 – 8

C) 1 – 6
   2 – 4
   3 – 7
   4 – 15
   5 – 2

K) 1 – 6
   2 – 5
   3 – 7
   4 – 8
   5 – 4

D) 1 – 2
   2 – 6
   3 – 2
   4 – 2
   5 – 1

L) 1 – 4
   2 – 3
   3 – 1
   4 – 2
   5 – 2

E) 1 – 2
   2 – 2
   3 – 2
   4 – 0
   5 – 2

M) 1 – 5
   2 – 1
   3 – 3
   4 – 3
   5 – 5

F) 1 – 12
   2 – 4
   3 – 12
   4 – 8
   5 – 6

N) 1 – 2
   2 – 5
   3 – 7
   4 – 5
   5 – 5

G) 1 – 2
   2 – 10
   3 – 8
   4 – 7
   5 – 10

O) 1 – 3
   2 – 3
   3 – 2
   4 – 4
   5 – 10

H) 1 – 4
   2 – 8
   3 – 4
   4 – 5
   5 – 5

P) Crisis Intervention—1
Promoting Employee Wellness—Nutrition/Exercise/Stress
Mgmt.—3
Aids Issue—5
Ethical & Moral Issues in Health Care & Prevention—3

Note: Only correctly completed surveys are included in these data.

catch up with you now. You will spend too much time analyzing data. You also might give your planning committee too much data so that you confuse rather than help the planning process.

REVIEWING AN EXAMPLE

A survey recently was used by the Community Health Programming Unit at the University of Wisconsin-Extension to assess the program-related needs of a varied adult target audience in a community of 50,000. The target populations included over 600 health and human service professionals, ministers, psychologists, guidance counselors, and teachers. A copy of the inventory is presented in Figure 3.1. By listing specific topics on the inventory, participants in the needs assessment were directed to respond to a delimited cluster of potential programming options. Had the inventory been completely open-ended, it could have been extremely difficult to detect a trend. Also, participants were further delimited to ranking only their top five choices. Participants did have the freedom to write in an option of their own, and then rank it. A few elected to do this.

The results of the survey are listed in Figure 3.2. For this tabulation, only those properly completing the survey were included. Another tabulation was made for those who incorrectly completed the survey. In comparing the two summaries, it was noted that many of the top-ranked issues correlated. The highest ranked issue on this survey was "Positive Self-Concept and Self-Esteem," followed by "Women/Men: Changing Roles," and then "Learning to Like Yourself." These final rankings were determined by changing the ranks into weighted values by multiplying the number of participants who rated a certain issue first, second, third, fourth, and fifth times the respective weight value (5, 4, 3, 2, 1). Thus, for "Positive Self-Concept and Self-Esteem," 12 respondents ranked it first, four ranked it second, 12 ranked it third, eight ranked it fourth, and six ranked it fifth, leading to weighted values of $(12\times5)+(4\times4)+(12\times3)+(8\times2)+(6\times1)$, and a total score value of 130.

4

Multi-Step Surveys - Delphi

INTRODUCTION

The Delphi Technique had its beginnings in the 1950s in a study done by the Rand Corporation for the United States Air Force. The study was aimed at using expert opinion to identify potential United States industrial targets and to estimate the number of atomic bombs needed to defend these targets against a Soviet attack. In 1964, the Delphi Technique was introduced to the larger scientific community when a study predicting the long-range trends in science and technology was released by the Rand Corporation (Linstone and Turoff, 1975). Since then, the Delphi has become a widely-used process in the areas of health, education, and social service.

The Delphi Technique is a form of group process that generates a consensus through a series of questionnaires. Usually the respondents are unable to meet in one place due to geographical or time limitations. Initially, the Delphi was developed as a forecasting technique, but is now used to clarify, prioritize, or identify problems and solutions. The process involves three groups: decision-makers, staff, and respondent group (Delbecq, et al., 1975, pp. 10, 85). In some organizations, the decision-makers and staff are the same group. The size of the respondent group varies, with 10 to 15 participants recommended for each representative group. A questionnaire consisting of one or two broad questions is sent out to the respondents. Their responses are analyzed and from these, a second questionnaire is developed. The respondents are asked to answer more specific questions for further clarification; their responses are again analyzed and another questionnaire is sent out asking for additional information. The process may end here or continue until there is a consensus. Usually, the number of rounds is three to five.

REVIEWING THE STRATEGY

Advantages of the Delphi Technique (Gilmore, 1977; Delbecq et al., 1975, pp. 34-35):

1. The Delphi is very responsive to subjective parameters and is therefore appropriate for situations when accurate information is not available.
2. People who are separated by geography or busy schedules can be in-

volved. This is especially useful when trying to obtain expert opinions.
3. There is no face-to-face contact, which reduces conformity, domination, or conflict.
4. Individuals who agree to participate in a Delphi study are usually highly motivated and committed, contributing a substantial amount of information.
5. The written response format encourages an increase in both the quality and quantity of ideas.
6. Participants' ideas are given equal representation through the synthesis.
7. The feedback process enables the participants to respond throughout the study and have a sense of closure when the study is completed.

Disadvantages of the Delphi Technique:

1. There is a large amount of administrative time and cost involved.
2. There is less opportunity to clarify the meaning of specific responses, which become open to the interpretation of the staff.
3. Since the participants do not meet directly, there is no opportunity for clarification of comments or further discussion on areas of disagreement. Points of disagreement are synthesized rather than addressed or resolved.
4. There is a considerable time commitment for the participants. Responding to the questionnaires may take up to 10 hours or more.
5. There are less rewards for the respondents, who must be inherently motivated to participate.

PREPARING FOR THE ASSESSMENT

At least 30 to 45 days should be allowed to prepare for the Delphi Technique. During this time the following tasks should be accomplished.

1. Develop a workgroup.
   The workgroup consists of staff and administrative people, usually five to nine members. They will develop and revise the questions, synthesize the responses, and determine the usefulness of the questionnaires.
2. Assign a coordinator.
   This person should be experienced in the Delphi technique, as well as knowledgeable about the problem being explored. This person will guide the workgroup.
3. Enlist ample support staff.
   You will need assistance in typing, mailing the questionnaires, and organizing the responses in a way that will facilitate the synthesis.

4. Establish a timeline.

A timeline will be very helpful in keeping the project on schedule.

5. Identify potential participants.

The workgroup or other people who are knowledgeable about the particular need area can generate a list or lists of people who can be contacted for their involvement in the Delphi. These potential participants should be interested in your topic, knowledgeable about the topic, and motivated to complete the series of questionnaires. Depending on the scope of your needs assessment, the list for each representative group can range from 25 to 100 people or more.

6. Clarify your goals and objectives.

If the decision-makers of your organization are not directly involved in the Delphi process, it is important to clearly understand what they want to accomplish. Clarification of goals and objectives will help structure the questions and organize the results of each questionnaire.

CONDUCTING THE ASSESSMENT

Once the preliminary steps are completed, you are ready to begin the Delphi process. Conducting the Delphi requires the following steps.

1. Develop the first questionnaire and pretest it.

This step is crucial. The question(s) must be understandable to the respondents and generate the kind of information you are seeking. Have several members of the staff or representative groups review the question(s) for any needed clarity.

The first questionnaire is generally broad in nature and simple in form, consisting of one or two open-ended questions, a request for a list with examples, or some other format that will generate information that is relevant and manageable for further questionnaires.

2. Choose the participants.

From the participant list or lists, individuals can be contacted and asked to nominate other respondents. Or, the individuals can be randomly selected from the list(s). A total of 10 to 15 people should be selected for each representative group. More people may be selected if you are working with only one homogeneous group, although this number should not exceed 30 (Delbecq, et al., 1975, p. 89). Once the respondents have been selected, they should be contacted in person, or by phone if this is not possible. They should be informed about the needs assessment, the purpose of the study, the make-up of the respondent group(s), the time investment and commitment required on the part of each respondent, and how the results will be shared.

3. Send out the questionnaire with a cover letter to the respondents. This should be done as soon as possible after the respondents have been contacted. Both the questionnaire and cover letter should be well-constructed and well-designed. Along with expressing appreciation for participating in the study, the cover letter should briefly outline the points that were presented in the initial contact with the participant. A response date of two weeks should be emphasized, and a stamped, self-addressed envelope should be enclosed for ease in responding.

   To encourage timely response, you may want to send out a letter or postcard in the second week, reminding the participants of the response date. A phone call also may be necessary for the late respondents.

4. Synthesize and analyze the responses of the first questionnaire. As the questionnaires are returned, the responses can be recorded on a master list for ease in analysis. Once all the questionnaires have been returned, call a meeting of the workgroup. Provide the members with a copy of the master list from which they can then sort the items into similar categories. Delbecq et al. (1975, p. 94) suggest listing each item on a 3x5 inch card and sorting them into piles of similar items. Then, each pile can be labeled and the labeled categories listed and discussed until there is a consensus among the group members upon a final list. The items in the final list then need to be summarized into clear and concise statements which will make up the second questionnaire.

5. Develop and send out the second questionnaire. The purpose of the second questionnaire is to get further clarification concerning the information from the first questionnaire. It should provide an accurate summary of the results of the first questionnaire. Participants are asked to review, comment, clarify, and vote on each specific item listed in the summary from the first questionnaire. The process of developing the second questionnaire should follow the same steps as the first questionnaire. The format employed will depend on the kind of information obtained from the first questionnaire and what kind of additional information is needed. Try to keep it short enough so that it can be completed in less than 30 minutes.

6. Synthesize and analyze the responses of the second questionnaire. The synthesis of the second questionnaire consists largely of a tally of the votes for each item. A tally sheet can be used that includes the list of items, the number of individuals voting for each item, the value of the individual votes, and the total vote. Comments should be summarized and then grouped with each item as in the first questionnaire.

7. If necessary, develop and send out a third questionnaire. Often, when a ranking of importance of each item is desired, a third questionnaire can be developed and sent out. This provides for addi-

tional consensus, as well as closure for the participants. The question-naire should be designed to enable the participants to review a sum-mary of previous comments and the results of the first vote for each of the items under consideration. A final ranking or vote plus any addi-tional comments can be requested. The procedure for developing and sending out the questionnaire is the same as for the previous questionnaires.

8. Synthesize and analyze the responses of the third questionnaire.
The responses of the third questionnaire can be summarized by tally-ing the final vote and incorporating additional comments into the pre-vious commentary.

USING THE RESULTS

Depending on the needs you are assessing, additional questionnaires may need to be developed and sent out to the respondents. The final questionnaire always should provide a prioritized list of items that can help in the planning process. The ranking of the items can indicate to the planners which items need to be addressed early in the planning process. When you have all the information you need, assemble the workgroup to review the data and develop a final report. The report should include a summary of all the questionnaires and recommendations for further planning based on the prioritization of the needs.

REVIEWING AN EXAMPLE

Representatives from the Department of Food Science at the Uni-versity of Wisconsin - Madison (Matthews, et al., 1975), in attempting to determine the future educational needs for administrative dietitians, used the Delphi Technique as a follow-up to a Nominal Group Process (to be described in Chapter 6). This follow-up measure was taken because it was considered impractical to reassemble the participants for another face-to-face meeting; however, issues raised at that meeting needed further refinement. In order to initiate the Delphi Process, they as-sembled a Delphi Analysis Group which developed the initial question-naire based on information from the Nominal Group Process. The 21 participants in the process included professionals involved in hospital food service, university faculty members, and students in dietetics. Three questionnaires at one-month intervals were mailed to the partici-pants. Responses from the first questionnaire were collated and summar-ized in order to develop the second questionnaire, and this process was then repeated for the final questionnaire. Each questionnaire was divided into three sections:

1. a list of major activities performed by the administrative dietitian (the results of ideas generated by the Nominal Group Process)
2. problems faced by the practicing dietitian which an entry-level dietitian should know how to solve. In responding to this section in the first questionnaire, the participants were asked to identify the problems and provide an example. In the second questionnaire, a 10-point rating scale was used (0 = "not important" and 10 = "extremely important"). The third questionnaire provided the participants with a compilation of the responses.
3. future professional activities of administrative dietitians. To address this section in the first questionnaire, one open-ended question encouraged the participants to think of the future role of administrative dietitians in 10 years and then identify and justify their major activities. For the second questionnaire, the Delphi Analysis Group formulated questions regarding the implications of the summarized participant responses. Ths third questionnaire provided a summary for the participants.

   The results of the overall process yielded valuable information for the staff regarding training and professional development needs for the administrative dietitian. Specified subject areas involved communication processes, problem-solving, evaluation, decision-making, and sanitation.

5

Interviewing

INTRODUCTION

If you like conversation, interviewing can be an exhilarating experience and a unique way to assess needs. Talking with people about their health needs, using the best interviewing techniques, can be as satisfying as planning a program based on those needs.

Interviews also can bring good results. People may resist completing another questionnaire, or refuse to participate in another telephone survey. They may be more agreeable to an interview, however, because it is a different experience. Most people like to talk about themselves. They feel flattered when selected to answer important questions. As a result, they may be primed to give you good information.

Conducting interviews, however, is not easy. The people you want to interview may be busy. They can be difficult to contact, to schedule an interview. When you do finally reach them, they may find it difficult to interrupt their activities to participate. Although people like to talk about themselves, they may resist talking about personal issues like health problems.

In spite of these challenges, interviews are a good way to assess needs. If you have the time and resources to conduct them, they can yield important information to use in planning educational and health promotional programs.

What is interviewing? A good interview is an exchange of information between two people: an interviewer, and an interviewee. It also may include emotional expression and persuasion, similar to a good conversation (Gorden, 1987, pp. 22-28). These characteristics are what make interviewing so fascinating. Not only do we obtain information from our interviewees, but we also learn their attitudes and their emotions.

Interviews can be formal or informal. Formal interviews can be highly scheduled, moderately scheduled, or nonscheduled. Highly scheduled interviews are similar to face-to-face and telephone surveys. (For specific information about highly-scheduled interviews, refer back to Chapter 3.) In this chapter we will focus on moderately scheduled and nonscheduled interviews conducted face-to-face. We will emphasize moderately scheduled interviews, since they are more frequently used to assess health needs.

Informal interviews are sometimes difficult to distinguish from ordinary conversation. The interviewer attempts to engage an individual in a conversation during which he or she is asked, for example, about some health-related issue. The interviewee may not recognize this exchange of information as an interview. The conversation may occur in a very informal setting, and typically is not arranged in advance. The interviewer will know what questions to ask, but will not refer to any notes, nor will the interviewer take any notes during the interview. As soon as possible thereafter, notes are written, typed, or dictated.

Informal interviewing may occur, for example, at a blood pressure screening site. An interviewer may ask people having their blood pressure checked how they feel about fluoridation of the community water supply. In this case the informal interview does not relate specifically to blood pressure screening. Instead the screening site is used to learn more about other health needs.

Although valuable insights can be gained from informal interviews, we will not describe them further. Since our focus is systematic needs assessment strategies, we will limit our discussion to formal interviews.

REVIEWING THE STRATEGY

Formal Interviews

Formal interviews are clearly identified as interviews. An individual is asked specifically to participate in an interview. The interviewer typically states the purpose of the interview, how the person has been selected to participate, and that responses will be treated confidentially. During the interview, the interviewer will refer to an interview schedule or guide and use some method of recording information.

A highly scheduled interview follows a very specific list of questions and instructions. The interviewer must proceed through these questions in exactly the same way for each participant. Background information and instructions to the participant are read verbatim from a script. Follow-up questions to clarify the meaning of responses and instructions on recording responses also are clearly specified.

At the other extreme, a nonscheduled interview gives the interviewer much more freedom and responsibility. The goals of the interview are specified, but the interviewer must decide what questions to ask and in what order. The interviewer also decides how to summarize the information received.

A moderately structured interview falls between these two extremes. The interviewer follows a set of questions, suggested follow-up questions, and instructions, but is free to use them differently during the interviews. The wording of the questions can vary, as well as the order in which they are asked. Additional follow-up questions can be asked if the interviewer believes they would yield helpful information. An interviewer need not ask all questions of each participant, if answers to those questions have already been obtained. Finally, the interviewer receives some guidance about summarizing the information but must decide what to include and what to omit. This variation from interview to interview is often appropriate when interviewing key informants.

Advantages of Moderately Scheduled Interviews

They offer more opportunity to discover information. Since a scheduled interview restricts the questions asked, the information obtained is restricted as well. A moderately scheduled interview gives the interviewer freedom to explore certain subjects more extensively with some participants than with others. Especially with key informants, the interviewer may pursue a particularly insightful response in great depth and discover important information not anticipated.

They offer the opportunity to obtain more complete information. The interviewer can ask as many follow-up questions as necessary to encourage participants to clarify and elaborate on their responses.

They are especially suited for obtaining valuable information from busy people. If necessary, the interviewer can focus on the questions that participants can answer most completely. By discussing in depth the areas they know best, the participants may feel they are using their time to its best advantage. If pressed for time, the interviewer can skip other questions.

Disadvantages of Moderately Scheduled Interviews

The interviewers need more knowledge of the subject of the interview. Since the interviewers make more judgments during the interview about what questions to ask and what questions to omit, knowledge of the subject is essential.

The interviewers need more extensive training. The interviewers need a complete understanding of the purpose of the interviews and more opportunities to conduct and critique practice interviews. They also need to practice recording and summarizing the information.

Data analysis is more difficult. Information obtained from highly scheduled interviews is primarily quantitative data. Moderately scheduled interviews yield primarily qualitative data. Analyzing this information requires more judgments about organization and interpretation.

They are more costly. Typically, more time is needed to complete a moderately-scheduled interview and record the information than with highly scheduled interviews. More time also is necessary to train interviewers and analyze data. Since the interviewers need a background in health education, they also may cost more to employ than a typical survey assistant.

These advantages and disadvantages also apply to *nonscheduled inter-*

views. The difference is one of degree. Since nonscheduled interviews place even more freedom and responsibility on the interviewer, they offer even more opportunity for discovery and in-depth information. Likewise, they require interviewers with more knowledge of the subject and more extensive training. Data analysis is even more difficult, and the complete process is more costly.

When deciding how extensively to structure the interviews for assessing health needs, consider the following questions.

1. Do you want to measure what all of your participants know about certain healthy behaviors? Or do you want to discover what needs might exist? The more you want to discover needs, the less you should structure the interviews.
2. Do you have interviewers with a background in health? The less background they have, the more structured your interviews must be.
3. How much time and money do you have for this project? The less you have, the more structured your interviews should be.

PREPARING FOR THE ASSESSMENT

To prepare for interviews, follow the same basic steps discussed for surveys in Chapter 3. However, how these steps are accomplished is different for interviews. One difference is the development of questions. Although drafting, testing, and modifying questions is important, it is not as critical to develop the ultimate questions. The interviewers exercise some judgment in how questions are asked during the interview. They can clarify the meaning of questions if participants are confused.

A second difference is the development of an interview schedule or guide. Telephone and face-to-face surveys call for a highly structured interview schedule. Moderately scheduled interviews, however, place more responsibility on the interviewer. They call for a list of questions to ask, along with suggested alternate wording and follow-up questions. The instructions need not be as specific nor the questions as precisely worded.

Another difference of interviews from surveys is the development of coding and data analysis procedures. Have some idea of how you plan to organize and analyze the data before you conduct the interviews. Try to anticipate the responses you are likely to receive and organize these anticipated responses into categories and general themes as best you can. This structure represents your best guess of how you will organize and eventually communicate the results of your interviews. It will be considerably less detailed than the coding and data analysis procedures developed for telephone and face-to-face surveys. It is also more tentative.

You can anticipate how you want to use the data, but you must always wait for the data you actually receive before committing yourself to a particular structure. The data may suggest other categories and themes which you could not anticipate before conducting the interviews. The less structured your interviews are, the less you can plan your coding and data analysis procedures before conducting your interviews.

Moderately scheduled and nonscheduled interviews, then, follow the same basic preparation steps as surveys. But, the time you save preparing for the interviews, you will spend after the interviews.

CONDUCTING THE ASSESSMENT

Many of the steps for conducting telephone and face-to-face surveys apply to conducting moderately scheduled or nonscheduled interviews. You must select a sample of people to interview, recruit and train your interviewers, and collect and record the data. How these steps are accomplished may vary considerably, depending on the interviews.

Select a Sample of Participants

The same systematic sampling procedures used for surveys may be appropriate for structured and non-structured interviews. The less structured the interviews are, however, the more you may want to interview certain key people. You also may want to interview fewer people, since data analysis will be a more extensive effort. You may place more importance on purposefully selecting specific people, rather than drawing a systematic sample.

You may decide to interview people who have the best perspective on the health needs of a particular community or organization. These key informants (Williams, 1978, p. 91) are selected because they can give you better information than you would obtain from a random sample. For a community they may be public health officials, health and human service professionals, school administrators, and leaders of religious organizations. Key informants in a private corporation can include the chief executive officer, senior managers, front line supervisors, personnel officers, and food service workers. (In such cases you do not claim to have selected a representative sample of a given population, but the individuals who can provide the best information.)

Develop a list of people to interview in priority order. This list should include more people than you need to interview. Some individuals will decline to participate, and others will be virtually impossible to contact.

Select and Train the Interviewers

Because moderately scheduled and nonscheduled interviews place more responsibility on the interviewers, you need to look for people who have both interviewing skills and a background in health education. Try to select individuals who are comfortable with and enjoy one-on-one, face-to-face situations. They should have the intelligence, flexibility, and emotional security to conduct a good interview (Gorden, 1987, pp. 207-209). The more background they have in health education and knowledge of the needs assessment project, the better. Knowledgeable interviewers have more credibility with interviewees, and can make informed judgments about follow-up questions to ask and leads to follow.

Extensive interviewer training is necessary for moderately scheduled and nonscheduled interviews. Similar to telephone and face-to-face surveys, the interviewers need to understand the purpose of the interviews, why they are important, and how the information will be used. They need instructions on contacting participants, handling ambiguous responses, and recording data. However, these interviewers need more information about the assumptions and philosophy which undergird the project. They also need more instructions about follow-up questions to ask and more opportunities to conduct and then critique practice interviews.

Devote at least one full day to interviewer training. After providing necessary background information and instructions, demonstrate a sample interview and have the group critique it. Then have each person conduct and critique one or two practice interviews on other interviewers. If possible, have each interviewer conduct at least one practice interview with a volunteer similar to those selected for the needs assessment. Have at least one other interviewer observe and then critique. These practice interviews also should include practice recording and summarizing data.

Collect and Record the Data

Telephone the individuals to arrange an appointment to conduct an interview. Since you will not reach everyone on the first try, decide in advance how many attempts to make before proceeding to contact someone else. State the purpose of the interviews, what organization is conducting them, why they are important, and how the information will be used. Explain how the individuals were selected to participate, and assure them that responses will be kept confidential. Then ask for an interview at a time and place convenient for the participants. Specify how long the interview will take. Interviewing key informants may require squeezing into their busy time schedules.

If possible, conduct the interviews in a place that has some association with your needs assessment. If you are interviewing health professionals about their needs for continuing education, offer to meet them in their offices or conference rooms. If you are interviewing consumers about their family eating patterns, offer to interview them in their homes. These locations make participation in the interview convenient, and they also help the individuals focus on the subject of the interview.

When conducting the interview, take a few moments to set the stage. Although the participants have been contacted by phone to set up the interview, they may have forgotten what was said or may not have been listening very closely. Repeat the same information about the project to refresh their memories. Emphasize confidentiality. Have them sign a consent form which gives permission to use the information obtained in the interviews.

The structure of the interview follows the same approach suggested for surveys in Chapter 3. Begin with questions that are relatively easy to answer. Ask potentially sensitive questions near the middle of the interview, and hold demographic questions until near the end. Interviewers should not refer to their interview schedule or guide as often as they would for a telephone or face-to-face survey. As much as possible, they should memorize the basic sequence of questions. Having the questions memorized allows them to concentrate on the interviewee and be more alert to following promising leads.

Remember that non-verbal cues are important for interviews. Gorden (1987, pp. 353-359) describes six non-verbal areas that affect the quality of the data: time, space, body movement, voice quality, touch, and smell. Arriving on time for the interview and concluding within the agreed-upon time elicits cooperation from the interviewees. But also give the participants enough space to communicate with a sense of freedom, and position yourself so you are talking one-on-one, as equals. Face the participants and use your posture to communicate a sense of relaxed anticipation; use good eye contact, nod, and smile appropriately; and use a tone of voice that is appropriate to each situation. Some participants may respond to a soft-spoken low-key interviewer. Other participants may need a more lively prodding to reveal good information.

Probing techniques are an essential part of interviewing. Probing involves the use of neutral prompts to persuade the interviewee to answer questions fully and completely. It is necessary when the interviewee offers no response at all or gives answers which are incomplete, irrelevant, poorly organized or unclear.

Probes are used to gain greater detail, elaboration, or clarification. Who, what, when, where, or how questions can encourage the interviewee to provide more detailed information. Gentle, approving nods and neutral comments ("yes, yes," "uh-huh") or questions ("Anything else?" "Then what?") are examples of elaboration probes. They are designed to keep the interviewee talking. Silence is also an effective elaboration probe. Resist the temptation to fill in gaps in the conversation. Let the interviewee do the talking as long as he or she has relevant information to offer. To clarify ambiguous, unclear, contradictory, or irrelevant answers, ask a neutral question ("What do you mean by that?" or "Why do you say that?"), or restate the original question to focus the interviewee's attention, or summarize what the interviewee has said so far to see if the interviewee will add more information. Finally, appearing puzzled may encourage the interviewee voluntarily to clarify the previous response. When probing, remember not to change the content or focus of a question, and watch the emphasis on words so as not to change the meaning.

Before concluding the interview, review the schedule or guide to ensure that all pertinent questions have been asked, especially if questions were asked in a different order from that listed on the schedule or guide. Lastly, thank the interviewee for participating, and conclude the interview promptly.

Recording data poses special challenges for moderately-scheduled or nonscheduled interviews. Unlike surveys, writing the responses in neat little boxes is not possible. Tape recording the interview is a possibility. A tape recording gives a complete record of the interview, which can be important for some interviews. However, some participants may feel inhibited by the presence of a tape recorder. More significantly, tape recordings require time and money to transcribe. Word-for-word transcriptions can take from two to six hours for every hour of interview time (Gorden, 1987, p. 263).

Most needs assessments do not require the same precision in recording data as rigorous academic research. An alternative to word-for-word transcription is to summarize the interview. Critical statements can be transcribed in their entirety; other statements can be condensed. Repetitive and unimportant statements can be ignored. This summary will take significantly less time to transcribe. It does require, however, a knowledgeable transcriber who can judge what to include and what to omit.

For most needs assessments, effective note taking during the interview is a good way to record data. This note taking is more difficult than for a survey. The questions are not as standardized, and the answers tend to be longer. However, the more structured the interview, the easier note taking will be. Capture the interviewee's own language as much as possible. Use direct quotes for essential statements or phrases. When extensive note taking is difficult during the interview, jot down key words or phrases. As soon as possible after the interview, preferably that same day, expand these notes into a more detailed summary of the interview.

USING THE RESULTS

What to do with the data following collection is a critical problem when using moderately-scheduled or nonscheduled interviews to assess needs. Talking with people about their needs can be an exhilarating experience. After the interviews are over, however, you have to make sense of the data stacked on your desk.

Using moderately-scheduled or nonscheduled interviews, most of the data collected will be qualitative. Now that you have the data, you need to decide whether pre-determined categories are still appropriate. Other categories may have become apparent during the interviewing. Use the questions asked during the interviews to suggest categories for data analysis, but stay open to other categories that emerge from responses of the participants. The more structured your interviews have been, the more your questions will remain appropriate as a way to organize your data. The less structured your interviews, however, the more you will need to develop another way to organize the data. Look for themes that are suggested by one or more of the categories. This exercise may require reading interview notes several times, developing a tentative structure, and refining that structure over a period of time.

In moderately-scheduled or nonscheduled interviews with key informants, you may not have asked everyone the same questions, so you cannot just count how many participants have expressed a certain need. You may have to present a narrative picture of the needs expressed. To do this, use case examples from the best responses to illustrate the needs you are describing. The less structured your interviews, the more this narrative picture is necessary.

Finally, consider how to present your findings to a planning committee or other interested groups. With a structured survey, you can rely heavily on a quantitative summary of the data and specific recommendations that follow. With moderately-scheduled and nonscheduled interviews, however, more responsibility rests on you to present and interpret the findings in a way that clearly represents the data.

REVIEWING AN EXAMPLE

Preliminary key informant interviews were used in a tri-county rural health promotion program development effort by the Institute of Man and Science in Rensselaerville, New York (Hanson, et al., 1983). These interviews provided basic information which was then complemented by additional strategies to include the community forum approach (described in Chapter 8). Those selected by the project team to serve as key informants included public health nurses, school teachers, social workers, health educators, mental health counselors, home health aides, cooperative extension agents, and clergy members. The interviews ranged in length from 45 minutes to two hours, and addressed the characteristics of the people served by the key informants, unmet health needs, procedures for skill development and information dissemination, potential for health education programming, and potential program obstacles.

The most frequently cited needs resulting from the summarized responses were the need for information about the recognition of health problems, decision-making skills related to medical care, referral sources for medical and screening services, support group and crisis assistance, conflict resolution education for parents, nutrition education, and school health instruction. Additionally, a few of the key informants suggested the development of a network of lay leaders in the tri-county villages to support the eventual efforts in health promotion.

Part III

Assessments with Groups

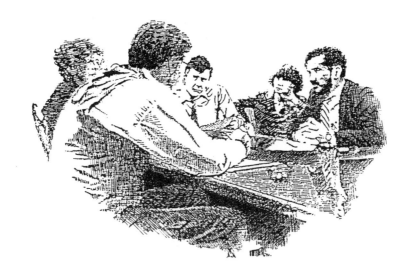

There are many ways to conduct needs assessments with assembled groups. In the next three chapters, we discuss the rather highly structured Nominal Group Process, as well as the less structured group processes of focus groups, community forum, participant observation, and electronic conferencing. These strategies often are coupled with other approaches to needs assessment in order to gain a more in-depth understanding of the reported needs.

6

Group Participation Process: Nominal Group

INTRODUCTION

The nominal group process was developed in 1968 by Delbecq and Van de Ven (1971; 1975) for assessments in business settings. It was based upon the involvement of a few target audience representatives in a highly structured process to qualify and quantify specific needs. Since its development, the process has been used by a variety of professionals, including those in health care, human service agencies, voluntary organizations, university extension, and educational settings (Bailey, 1973; Gilmore, 1977; Van de Ven and Delbecq, 1971).

The nominal group process utilizes groups of five to seven people who have some knowledge of the issues being examined. Group members are asked to write responses to a question, without discussing it among themselves. Then, each participant shares one of his or her responses in a round-robin fashion which continues until every response from each individual is recorded. The responses are clarified through discussion. The participants then select and rank a stated number of items which they think are the most important. The process may stop at this point or there may be a discussion of the preliminary vote followed by a final vote.

REVIEWING THE STRATEGY

Though not a great deal of reading is required of the participants, clear and concise writing ability by the representatives greatly aids the process. Group involvement and understanding of health issues are important requirements of the representatives. The nominal group process provides both quantitative data in the sense of voted-upon priorities, and qualitative data in terms of a descriptive discussion of the problem (Delbecq et al., 1975, pp. 4-10). The qualitative data flow from the discussion, which is characteristic throughout most of the nominal group process. Members often provide critical incidents or personal anecdotes. The combined qualitative and quantitative data encourage professional reaction to client needs.

One of the difficulties planners face when using the nominal group process is finding people who are willing to commit over an hour of their time to the process. You may want to elicit participation by invitation— either of specific people or in an open situation in which people can reply with a commitment to participate. You also may seek cooperation from groups already in existence.

Advantages of the Nominal Group Process

1. It allows direct involvement of the service population. Those who may be most affected by a particular problem can be actively involved in its identification and scope.
2. There is an equal opportunity for all participants to share their ideas and be actively involved.
3. Because of the disciplined process, minority opinions and conflicting ideas are tolerated. The process attempts to avoid the evaluation of the ideas until the very end, when voting takes place.
4. The process avoids arguments over semantics and wording through a clarification step.
5. Since everyone is given an opportunity to write down their ideas first and then discuss, all are encouraged to participate. This also tends to reduce the potential for control or use of hidden agendas by one or two participants.
6. The nature of the group process—especially since it encourages writing down ideas and discussion—generates a creative tension and stimulates more ideas.

Disadvantages of the Nominal Group Process

1. Because of the amount of time required, there may be scheduling problems or difficulty finding participants willing to commit over an hour of their time.
2. The group responses may deviate from the intended direction of the written questions and participants may end up focusing on an issue different from the original.
3. Biases can enter into the nominal group process since it encourages personal opinions, beliefs, and experiences.
4. Often the people who identify the need have no further involvement in the continuing program planning process.

PREPARING FOR THE ASSESSMENT

Four to eight weeks before conducting the Nominal Group Process, you should complete much preliminary work.

1. Identify potential groups for participation.
   Ask yourself which specific populations make up your target audience during a particular programmatic phase (for example, health education for primary prevention through immunizations), or time period. Next, consider what size of a sample of the target audience would

reflect that group's needs, and identify specific people who can make up that sample by being invited to a nominal group meeting.

2. Enlist and train facilitators.

Attempt to have a facilitator for each grouping of five to seven people. Explain to the facilitators the purpose of the nominal group process and the specific steps they will be following. Also, have them assist you in the development of the question to be posed to the representatives.

To fully prepare facilitators for the various details related to the process, we recommend taking them through a trial run as participants. Compose a question and then move the facilitators through the entire process. Following the entire experience, allow time for specific questions about the process. Emphasize the need for preplanning, particularly in regard to arrangement of facilities and materials.

3. Develop the question.

The question you develop must be clear and simply stated. Delbecq et al. (1975, pp. 66; 75-77) have emphasized that the question should be generated after considering (a) the objective of the meeting, (b) example of the type of items sought, (c) the development of alternative questions, and (d) the pilot-testing of alternative questions with a sample group. A planning committee can be very helpful during this part of the process. One example of a question is: "What do you consider to be the major health problems you are facing at this time?" This type of question can be placed at the top of a sheet of paper and copied to hand out to the participants.

4. Arrange the facilities and materials.

Consider where to hold a meeting of your representatives. You may find that it is best to hold several meetings at different locations for the convenience of the target audience. We have used this approach in multi-county assessments. The following materials will be needed: one chalkboard, flipchart, or other large writing surface per small group; 3 x 5 inch cards (allow 10 to 18 cards per person); a sheet of paper stating the group questions; pencils; and an information sheet to collect demographic data. The facilities you need include a large meeting room with space for smaller groups of five to seven people. The rooms should be equipped with tables or desks and should be comfortable. If it is necesary to use the large room for several smaller groups, try to keep the groups as separate as possible so the work of one group does not influence or hinder other groups.

CONDUCTING THE ASSESSMENT

Using the Nominal Group Process, follow these steps to conduct the assessment.

1. Convene as a large group.
   Explain the purpose of the meeting and the process which will be used. Establish a comfortable environment.
2. Arrange the participants into groups of five to seven members, and assign a facilitator to each group. It is important that the size of each group does not exceed seven, to allow for appropriate interaction. Those selected as participants should be representative of, and knowledgeable about, the community in question. The facilitator introduces himself/herself and emphasizes the need for full participation. It is important to keep in mind that the nominal group process is designed to encourage everyone to participate openly without being impeded or overwhelmed by the titles of others in the group. (We have found it helpful for the participants to introduce themselves *without* stating their positions of employment.)
3. Pose a single question to the group, and have the participants write down their responses. It is best if the question can be in writing on a chalkboard, flipchart, or handout sheets. (We have found that handouts are the easiest for the participants to use since it keeps the question in front of them and provides space to write responses.) Sheets of paper with the question listed at the top can be given out; this provides an easy reference point for the group members. However, if this is not possible, writing the question down on a chalkboard, flipchart, or overhead projector will suffice.
   Although the actual amount of time necessary to write the responses will vary, depending upon the particular question, an approximate amount of time would be 15 minutes. It is important that the group proceed in absolute silence. (This is the responsibility of the group leader.) Such an approach enables each member to reflect carefully upon his or her own ideas, to be motivated by the observance of others who are working diligently by writing down their responses, and to be involved in a competition-free atmosphere where premature decisions do not have to be made.
4. Elicit individual responses in a round-robin fashion.
   One participant begins by giving a single response, the next gives a single response, and this continues until each participant has contributed a single response. As the responses are stated, they are written by the group leader on a chalkboard or flipchart, each item being numbered. The same process is repeated until all contributions have been recorded. This procedure enables each group member to fully participate. During this time, there is no discussion permitted regarding form, format, or meaning of a participant's response.
5. Clarify the meaning of the responses.
   Take time to be certain each response is clearly understood. Allow participants time to discuss what they meant by a particular response,

the logic behind it, and its relative importance. However, this is not the time for argumentation and lobbying. The group leader must direct the proceedings so that only clarification takes place.

6. Conduct and discuss a preliminary vote.

From the original listing of responses, participants are directed to select and rank a stated number of the items they consider the most important. This is accomplished by writing each one of the statements on a separate card, and then rank-ordering them. Delbecq, et al. (1975, p. 58) point out that group members can prioritize only five to nine items with some degree of reliability. Participants are asked to list the item number along with the statement in the upper left-hand portion of the card. When all the participants have accomplished this for the statements they have selected, they should rank the cards by placing the rank number in the lower right-hand portion of the card and underlining it.

On the chalkboard (or flipchart), the group leader then records the rankings assigned to the statement selected by each participant and sums up the votes after all participants have contributed their rankings. The item with the largest numerical total represents the top priority issue. Note: In most instances, this completes the process. However, in order to increase the level of accuracy, it can be extended to include discussing the vote or conducting another vote (see steps 7 and 8).

Discuss the various explanations related to the voting patterns. Discussion regarding the high vote-getters and low vote-getters may be of value. It also may be useful to redefine the meaning of selected items, to be certain that all participants are clear on their meaning.

7. Conduct a final vote.

For this step, two procedures can be used: (a) as followed in the preliminary vote, select a stated number of the most important items, and then rank-order them; or (b) select a stated number of the most important items, and then rate them. To rate them, if there are seven major items selected, each one of them could be rated on a scale of zero (not important) up to 10 (very important). This procedure then provides insight regarding the actual magnitude of differences between the major items.

8. Calculate the total vote.

Remembering that there may be several groups of representatives completing this process, it is important to calculate a grand total vote. First, the items from all of the groups are arranged into similar categorical areas (as closely as possible), and then the numbers from rank-ordering or rating are added together in each categorical area. For example, if three items from group one, two items from group two, and four items from group three relate to health problems with rodent infestation, the total value (from ranking or rating) is calculated for all nine items. The resulting value is then listed for the categorial need area of "Health problems related to rodent infestation." As the total votes are calculated for each categorical area, it will be realized that they can be placed in descending order. The categorical area with the largest number is considered to be of the highest priority.

9. Compile and prioritize the data.

Once the data are compiled for each group, the next task is to combine similar need areas and the ratings (see Tables 6.1 and 6.2). Similar specific needs from each group are assimilated into a combined need statement. Also, the individual ratings for each specific need are combined (see step 2 in Table 6.1). Finally, general need areas are established and aligned with a grouped rating value for each area, with the combined and general need areas. The quantitative analysis relates to the final rating values.

Needs assessed through the nominal group process are carefully re-

Table 6.1. *Nominal Group Process: Organizing the Data.*

1. Plot Group Results (for given geographical area)

Group I		Group II		Group III	
Specific Need	Final Rating	Specific Need	Final Rating	Specific Need	Final Rating
Item A	40	Item A	2	Item A	28
B	33	B	15	B	7
C	0	C	17	C	19
D	50	D	28	D	44
E	2	E	48	E	12
F	19	F	41	F	22
G	21	G	3	G	37
H	33	H	0	H	18
I	5	I	29		
J	16	J	35		
		K	21		
		L	38		
		M	9		

NOTE: These are *specific* need priorities.

2. Combine *Similar Specific* Needs and Their Ratings

Example: Item D (Group I) + Item F (Group II)

+ Item H (Group III) =

	Specific Need	Final Rating
	Combined Need Statement	109

Table 6.2. *Nominal Group Process: Establishing General Need Areas.*

(Rank)	Final Rating
1. General Need Area No. 1	221
a. Combined specific need area	109
b. Specific need area	44
c. Specific need area	35
d. Specific need area	33
2. General Need Area No. 2 (Follow same procedure)	

NOTE: May have to use "miscellaneous" and "unclassifiable" categories as general need areas.

viewed by the planning committee. While the qualitative and quantitative data presented in Table 6.2 appears quite absolute, one should not be guided solely on this tabular arrangement. Consider the commentary of your planning committee regarding additional needs that may not have been directly stated, but rather implied; consider potential reformulations of the general and combined need areas; and consider potential resources and barriers in addressing each one of the identified needs. Then, have the planning committee establish the final priority listing.

USING THE RESULTS

One particular advantage resulting from the nominal group data compilation is that you have a quantified summary of the group discussion. This can be used in your planning process as one source of information. However, make certain to remind your planning committee that this is not to be construed as the end result of an explicit research process, but rather the summary of a group interaction process. Inform them that the numbers are not absolutes. Whether or not you choose to address those needs with the highest priority listing will depend on multiple factors, such as lead time, available resources, target audience readiness, and the opportunity for success. For example, you initially may wish to address a lower priority need because of available resources and the high chances for success. Where and when you start can be a planning committee decision.

REVIEWING AN EXAMPLE

The nominal group process was selected by health professionals to assess health-related needs in the rural community of Bloomer, Wisconsin (Bailey, 1973). A total of 225 out of approximately 3,200 residents participated in 30 nominal group meetings over a three-month period. In response to the question, "What more do you need to know about the health of you and your family to be physically and mentally fit?," 529 health needs were identified. After indexing the needs in accordance with the Medical Subject Heading classification system of the National Library of Medicine, 25 prioritized health-related listings emerged. The top five in descending order were, Drug, Alcohol, Tobacco Addiction; Health Manpower; Family Living; Health Care Delivery System; and Emergency Care and Safety. Each classification was further subdivided into prioritized categories, later reviewed and addressed by the planning committee.

The health professionals using this process felt that it enabled the residents' needs to evolve, resulting in a richer source of information; that this was a reasonable procedure for a community setting since it did not lock people into preconceived goals; that the process was effective in determining perceived health education needs; and any inadvertent staff bias was kept to a minimum. There also was the suggestion that the process would serve to motivate the community members to meet their own selected health needs.

7

Group Participation Process: Focus Group

INTRODUCTION

The focus group has its roots in the group depth interview that was developed as a form of group therapy (Boyd, et al., 1981; Churchill, 1979). In the 1950s, the technique was borrowed from psychiatry and developed as a marketing research technique (Bellenger et al., 1976; Gage, 1980). It is in this area that the focus group has gained prominence. Today it is one of the most widely used marketing research techniques, expanding into other areas, including government and social change organizations (Antilla and Sender, 1982).

The focus group is typically an exploratory process that is used for generating hypotheses, uncovering attitudes and opinions, and acquiring and testing new ideas. It utilizes groups of six to 12 people that are fairly homogeneous in nature. The groups gather in a relaxed, informal setting to participate in an unstructured interview. A moderator has the task of focusing the group on the discussion topic and skillfully guiding the discussion in a way that stimulates interaction and encourages the sharing of feelings, attitudes, and ideas from all group members. Usually the discussion is tape-recorded or video-taped; if facilities are available, the focus group process can be viewed by administrative staff through a one-way mirror or closed-circuit television.

REVIEWING THE STRATEGY

Advantages of the Focus Group:

1. It is a relatively inexpensive method of using an exploratory approach to assess needs.
2. It is easy to arrange and can be completed in a short amount of time.
3. Because of the ease of implementation, a larger number of homogeneous groups, or more diverse groups, may be involved in this process than in other needs assessment strategies.
4. The group process stimulates a wide range of ideas, emotions, and information. A comment from one person may stimulate ideas, feelings, or opinions from other people in the group. These comments are accepted as valuable information.
5. The focus group structure enables the moderator to obtain clarification if needed.

6. The lack of rigid structure allows for the free exchange of feelings, ideas, attitudes, perceptions, and thoughts. It encourages spontaneity and open, honest expression.
7. Unlike the nominal group process, there is greater tolerance to deviate from the intended direction and to explore related ideas and concerns. Deviations are analyzed as carefuly as other responses. However, it is the moderator's job to direct the group back to the topic if the discussion becomes irrelevant.

The focus group is limited by the following disadvantages:

1. The data are exclusively qualitative, making coding, tabulating, and analyzing difficult (Churchill, 1979).
2. Sample sizes are quite small and randomization of the sample may be limited. Results are not easy to generalize.
3. The results are dependent on the skill of the moderator. An inexperienced moderator or a moderator who has preconceived ideas can produce misleading results.
4. The information obtained from focus groups cannot stand alone. It is unwise to make decisions based solely on focus group results. Additional assessment should be done before making decisions.
5. Recruitment of participants may be difficult, especially when trying to identify homogeneous groups in a short amount of time.
6. Depending on the skill of the moderator, some participants may not have an equal chance of participating. Some individuals may dominate the interaction, not allowing the more shy individuals an opportunity to participate.

PREPARING FOR THE ASSESSMENT

Some market researchers have assembled a focus group within minutes. However, a little planning one to two months prior to the focus group discussion will help to focus the entire project.

1. Develop an interview guide.
   The interview guide outlines the scope of the need area that you will be assessing. Its purpose is to assist the moderator in introducing the topic or topics and focusing on these areas as needed throughout the discussion.
2. Enlist a well-trained, experienced moderator.
   The moderator is a crucial part of the focus group process. He or she must have good interpersonal communication skills and be able to quickly establish rapport and gain the confidence of the participants (Zikmund, 1982). Ideally the moderator should fit in with the group. For example, if working mostly with women, the moderator should be

a woman. This is not always possible, especially when using a diversity of groups. The same moderator should be used for all groups (Bellenger, et al., 1976). Familiarize the moderator with the goals and objectives of the needs assessment, as well as the mission, philosophy, and operations of your organization (if the moderator is from outside your organization). Be sure you and the moderator become acquainted before beginning the focus group process (Miskovic, 1980).

3. Determine the number and makeup of the groups.

A rule of thumb is to continue conducting focus groups until no new ideas are generated. This generally occurs after three or four groups (Boyd, et al., 1981). You may want to conduct more focus groups, depending on the kind of information you are seeking, the diversity of your groups, and time and cost allowances. If you want information from people of different backgrounds, you should identify those subgroups and conduct three to four groups for each subgroup. Never use only one focus group.

The makeup of the groups should be as homogeneous as possible. This reduces variations in responses based on social, intellectual, lifestyle, or demographic differences. People of similar backgrounds are more likely to relate better to one another and this will enhance the focus group discussion.

4. Select participants.

Establish "quotas" for participants based on criteria that will produce the most homogeneous groups. These quotas may include gender, age, income, education, or other demographic factors that may affect how people respond to the need area (Boyd, et al., 1981). For example, you may want to separate mothers who work outside the home from those who do not when assessing needs for health care services for children. The perceptions of these two groups may be significantly different and interfere with participants' abilities to relate to each other. Putting them together in one focus group may hinder the discussion.

Participants may be recruited from ads, lists, or other means using the quotas to screen the most appropriate candidates. They should have adequate background or experience so they can contribute to the discussion. The participants should not know each other prior to the meeting since this may influence group interaction. However, this is not always possible to achieve in small communities. In these situations at least try to avoid placing close friends in the same group. The participants should not have been in a similar group interview for at least six months (Bellenger, et al., 1976). Sometimes participants are paid for their involvement.

5. Arrange the facilities.

Where the focus group is held is important to the success of the process. The setting should be very relaxed and informal. Sometimes it is appropriate to meet in the home of one of the participants. Avoid meeting around a large conference table which is usually too large and formal to create a comfortable environment. The site of the focus group may be influenced by what type of recording is being done. Use of a one-way mirror or closed-circuit television will require more specific facilities, whereas tape-recording or videotaping allows for more selectivity in choosing the meeting site. The most critical factors are that the room be comfortable to allow for open communication and that it be easily accessible to the participants.

CONDUCTING THE ASSESSMENT

1. Allow time for participants to gather and talk among themselves. This gives them an opportunity to get to know each other and become more comfortable with the surroundings. The moderator introduces him or herself and then asks the participants to introduce themselves. Participants also can be asked to share with the group something about themselves that relates to the topic. For example, if the need area concerns children and you are meeting with young parents, you may want to ask them to tell the group something about their children.
2. The moderator introduces the process and the topic. The moderator provides a brief description of the process and offers some guidelines for the discussion: speak so that everyone can hear; speak one at a time; and be open and honest in expressing what you think and feel, whether it be positive or negative (Luck, et al., 1982).

    The moderator then makes some general comments about the purpose of the meeting, being careful not to imply any expectations. He or she then makes a statement or asks a question that will open the discussion.
3. The moderator carefully guides the discussion. Once the moderator initiates the discussion, the group is free to interact with each other in pursuing the topic. The moderator takes a less dominant role in the group, getting involved only to ask questions that will keep the discussion moving, to introduce a new dimension to the topic, or to refocus the group if it has completely lost track of the topic. The moderator must carefully direct the discussion in a way that both maintains optimum freedom of the group interaction and elicits information that is relevant to the need area. In order for the moderator to focus on the group interaction, taping is strongly recommended. Trying to record notes about the event while it is happening will result in missed data. If

only audio taping is available, the moderator may want to make some notations on nonverbal behaviors throughout the interview.

4. If the process is being directly observed by other staff through a one-way mirror or closed-circuit television, they should keep in mind the following points: Realize that what is being watched is work in progress. Listen actively and selectively, rather than for what you want to hear. Watch for non-verbal cues. Trust the moderator; however, if the process is not going well, speak up (Miskovic, 1980).

5. Bring the discussion to a close.
   When all the areas outlined in the guide have been addressed, the discussion can be brought to a close. The moderator should ask the participants to offer a summary of what was discussed and what was resolved.

6. After several days, a follow-up call can be made to all participants to thank them for their involvement. You also may ask for any additional information and ideas they may have generated since the focus group meeting (Bellenger et al., 1976).

USING THE RESULTS

Following each focus group, the moderator should meet with you to clarify what occurred in the session. A transcript should be made from the audio or videotape and then synthesized, analyzed, and interpreted. Bernstein (1978) suggests that the information is more significant if the people in the focus group became quickly involved without much prodding from the moderator, if the participants used the first person instead of the third person, or if they indicated some past experiences with this need area. Consider these points as you develop the report. The report should be written to include the following: implications, interpretations, hypotheses, theories of how things are or could be, and recommendations (Miskovic, 1980). The report should be integrated with quantitative and other qualitative data before making any decisions related to program planning.

REVIEWING AN EXAMPLE

In 1985, Keller et al. (1987) conducted focus group assessments with 22 individuals 65 years of age and older (senior citizen group), and 16 individuals 22 to 40 years of age (baby boom group) in the midwest. Their purpose was to assess the beliefs and needs of the senior citizen population from the vantage point of both groups. The process employed a qualitative approach in attempting to observe and understand phenomena and situations in their entirety, leading to the eventual generation of hypotheses.

Four focus groups assessments were conducted in two communities, the groups ranging from seven to 13 participants. Of the two senior citizen groups, one was held in a senior citizen center and one in a high-rise; the two baby boom groups were hosted by a real estate agency and at a participant's residence. The group moderator used nine questions during the process, addressing, for example, words or phrases which describe senior citizens, positive aspects about growing old, senior citizen health status, and special needs of the elderly. Additionally, a questionnaire was used to obtain demographic data, and follow-up telephone calls sought reactions to the process and any additional ideas. The comments were tape recorded (with permission) and transcribed in order to retain the full meaning expressed by the participants.

The responses were organized into nine categories aligned with the questions, with preferences and non-preferences by each group noted. Agreements between the groups (for example, more positive ratings of health status and more positive patient/physician relationships) were reported by the senior citizen group. Overall, Keller et al. (1987) found the process useful in eliciting age-related beliefs and stimulating participant expression in order to get at the how and why of those beliefs.

8

Other Group Assessment Processes

INTRODUCTION

Two very specific and popular group needs assessment strategies were addressed in Chapters 6 and 7. There are several additional strategies which can offer insight into group needs. These include the community forum (also referred to as the public hearing), participant observation as a non-reactive group assessment, and electronic conferencing.

COMMUNITY FORUM
Reviewing The Strategy

The community forum approach to assessing needs (sometimes referred to as a public hearing) is an attempt to identify needs of communities and neighborhoods through public meetings. While the main effort at these meetings is to inform the public, they also can seek the need-related insights of those in attendance. Witkin (1984, p. 130) noted that a variety of formats can be used in the community forum: hearings enabling people to speak as long as they desire; meetings in which each speaker has a limitation on the amount of speaking time; meetings which use a group survey, asking participants to rank or rate statements or respond to questions; and the small group approach in which participants are divided into small groups for discussion and eventual feedback to the total group. Typically, the community forum approach is used to identify general need areas which are later refined through additional strategies.

A community forum is a public meeting which invites participation from anyone in the community wishing to offer his or her perspective on a particular issue. It seeks to involve a broad cross-section of the community in order to review various points of view. In some cases a community forum is conducted by a unit of local government as a public hearing, following the statutes governing that unit. Other times, a community forum is conducted less formally.

The advantages of a community forum are:

1. A community forum is relatively straightforward to conduct. People are invited to come to a community facility to express their views on an issue one at a time; you record what they say. Compared to a nominal group process, for example, it is much simpler to run and requires fewer staff members with less extensive training.

2. A community forum is relatively inexpensive. The only costs are for publicity, staff time to attend the forum, staff time to record and analyze the information gathered from the forum, and possibly rental fees for the facility used.
3. Because the forum is publicly advertized, it offers the opportunity to hear the views of all segments of the community.
4. People can participate on their own terms. They can come to the forum and simply state what is on their minds. They do not have to master a certain technique or follow a structured set of questions.
5. A community forum can help identify people from the community who are most interested in addressing the determined needs. The people who take the time to participate in a forum are likely those who feel most strongly about the issues and want to see them addressed. They are people who may later be involved in planning ways to meet the identified needs.

The disadvantages of a community forum are:

1. It is often difficult to get good attendance. Although a forum usually has the potential to attract a cross-section of the community, in reality it rarely does. As a result, the people who do participate will offer only a partial view of the needs that exist.
2. Participants in the community forum tend to be those representing special interests. They are the ones with the most to gain or lose, so they usually are the ones who are most motivated to come. People with less of an investment in the issue may have valuable insights to offer, but because they are not as highly motivated, they may not take the time to come. Therefore, although the participants in a community forum may be good candidates for helping to meet the identified needs later on, they also may represent special interests which can skew the planning process.
3. The forum could possibly degenerate into a gripe session. Since the format allows people to say what is on their minds, they may avoid focusing on particular needs to be addressed. While other strategies for needs assessment can be more difficult for the participants to relate to, they do introduce some structure which can prevent the process from becoming a gripe session.
4. Data analysis can be time consuming. Since the information gathered from a community forum may not follow any particular pattern, it will be necessary to develop a structure after the forum and determine the best way of summarizing and presenting the findings.

The best way to consider the role of a community forum in the needs assessment process is as a test of needs which have been identified through some other process. Needs which have been identified can be presented to the public through the forum to determine whether the public confirms them as needs. It is a way of legitimizing needs which have been identified, as well as allowing new needs to surface.

Preparing For The Assessment

1. Develop one or more questions which the forum will address. It is better to use questions rather than a general topic, since the participants will have an opportunity to focus their comments. It also makes it easier for them to respond, and may increase their motivation to participate.

2. Determine how many forums to schedule. There are several criteria to keep in mind when determining how many forums to conduct. If you want to obtain the broadest possible participation, you may need to schedule several forums at different times and in different places. If you want to draw people from a wide geographical area, then you will want to schedule them to minimize travel distances. Keep in mind the type of people you want to come. An evening forum usually will be necessary in order to attract working people, but may discourage elderly people from attending. They may need the opportunity to attend a forum during the day. A final criterion is the amount of time and money you have to complete your needs assessment. Although a community forum is relatively inexpensive, each forum does involve certain costs.

3. Schedule the forum or forums in accessible places. Often a well known public facility located in a convenient location works well (a public library, city hall, local school, or community center). Even hospitals and colleges can be used if they are known for their community service work. When scheduling the facility, consider the availability of parking at the time the forum will be held.

4. Publicize the forum widely. Take advantage of as much free publicity as possible from the mass media. Send press releases to local daily and weekly newspapers, radio stations, and television stations. Follow up these news releases by contacting news reporters and try to arrange an appointment to discuss the importance of the upcoming forum and encourage the release of an article in advance of the forum. Try to arrange to be interviewed by radio and television reporters and participate in call-in talk shows or local community features if possible.

Do not rely solely on the mass media, however, to publicize the forum. Consider mailing flyers to organizations interested in the issues to be addressed, and ask these organizations to publicize the forum to their members (perhaps by placing an announcement in their newsletters). Place notices in widely-used public sites such as public libraries, banks, restaurants, and supermarkets. If your budget permits, you may want to mail letters or flyers directly to individuals or groups you especially want to attract to the forum.

In the publicity materials for the forum, make sure to specify what participants will be asked to do. Clearly identify the question or questions they should address. Give them the opportunity to speak at the forum and to submit written commentary if desired.

5. Make the necessary on-site arrangements; make sure there are enough chairs. Typically, the staff would be seated at a table slightly removed from the participants, with paper and pens to take notes as desired. If the room is large, microphones should be provided both for the participants and for the staff members who may wish to ask questions. A staff member should register the participants as they arrive and receive any written materials they wish to submit. Be sure the room is well-marked both outside and inside the building. If the budget permits, providing light refreshments can contribute to a congenial gathering.

Conducting the Assessment

1. Start the forum on time. The person conducting the forum should welcome the participants, thank them for coming, introduce him or herself and the other staff members, briefly state the purpose of the forum, and explain how the event will be conducted.
2. Keep the forum moving. Invite the participants to participate in the order in which they registered upon arrival, unless you have in mind some other plan for the order of presenting comments.
   Encourage the participants to keep their remarks within the allotted time, typically five or 10 minutes. After the participant comments, allow each staff member present to ask the participant any questions for clarification or follow-up. Usually, you will not want to have your staff or members of the audience engage in a discussion of what was said. The purpose of a forum is to allow everyone an opportunity to speak in an orderly fashion, with opportunities for clarification by staff members.
3. Conclude the forum when appropriate. It is difficult to predict what will happen during a community forum. If only a few people show up, there will be more opportunity to ask questions of the participants. If a large crowd attends, it may be best to restrict the follow-up questions to keep the forum from dragging on too long. Thank the people for their participation and assure them that their commentary will be used in planning to address the needs identified.

Using the Results

As noted earier, it is difficult to structure the data analysis until after the forum. Analyzing the data from a community forum can be similar to analyzing the data from key informant interviews, as explained in Chapter 5. Read through the information to determine what categories emerge and then summarize the data under each one of these categories. Again, a community forum may be best used to confirm needs determined by other needs assessment strategies. Compare the needs that surfaced from the forum with these other needs before making final decisions about needs to be addressed.

PARTICIPANT OBSERVATION

Reviewing the Strategy

Health professionals sometimes place themselves in group situations for varying amounts of time in order to gain a sense of group health needs. Examples include attending a community group's series of meetings as a known representative of a health agency without serving in any official capacity, or attending such meetings as a concerned citizen with one's professional responsibilities undeclared. In both examples, the health professional attempts to accumulate visual and auditory cues which eventually may lead to clear patterns of an expressed need. However, no matter how well integrated into the group this person becomes, there may be an inherent bias interjected into the group discussions and interactions due to that person's presence. (Webb et al., 1966, p. 113).

Advantages of participant observation are:

1. Participant observation enables one to observe the unique interaction of group members directly, rather than serving necessarily as an outside observer.
2. Typically, there is a minimum of outside interference (e.g., activities of other groups) as one views the selected group members working together in their natural environment.
3. Typically, there is built-in flexibility with the observation timeframe to allow for a observation at a series of group meetings. This provides several opportunities to examine trends over time, and, if necessary, have them clarified and corroborated by certain group members.
4. There is flexibility in the information-gathering procedures so that one does not feel "locked in" to a single process during one event.

Disadvantages of participant observation are:

1. There is potential for the observer to exert (knowingly and unknowingly) some influence on the discussion patterns and decisions, and observer inclination for only certain types of information (Webb and Weick, 1983).
2. Participant observation is a time-consuming activity. In addition to the time spent sitting through an entire meeting, you have to allow

travel time to and from the meetings, and time (very soon after the meeting) to commit your observations to writing.

3. Attendance at more than one meeting of the group is usually necessary. Unlike a nominal group process or a community forum, which are very structured group meetings designed to yield very specific information in one meeting, participant observation is much more unpredictable and open-ended. Although one meeting can yield much information about health-related needs, the following two or three meetings may provide little information. Due to the time and staff resources which need to be committed to such a venture, determine whether or not the benefits will be worth the cost.

Preparing for the Assessment

1. Determine what specifically you are looking for. If there are very specific questions about health-related needs you want to try to answer from observing a group, be very focused in your observations, paying particular attention to those group interactions which help answer those questions. More often, however, you may not have such a sharply-focused list of questions. In that case, you will want to pay attention to a wider range of group interactions. Also, determine the scope of your participant observation activities. Determine how many groups are to be observed, how many meetings of each group to attend, and how active you want your observers to be during these group meetings.

2. Select your observers. The participant observer may be yourself, or you may need additional observers if you plan to observe more than one group. More significantly, however, you may decide in some situations that you are not the best person to observe the group. Many of the group members may know you, and you may believe this relationship will unduly bias the group interaction. In those situations, it may be best for the observer to be someone they do not know. Also, your professional status may be a hindrance to the group. Then, it may be advisable to recruit people who can more easily blend in with the group members. Just as good teaching is often considered an art, so is good participant observation; some people are more naturally gifted.in this area than others. Thus, in the observer selection process, consider whether individuals have the personality to become good observers, and how much experience they have had working with groups.

3. Train the observers. Explain the purpose of the observation to your observers and tell them what to look for. Discuss good techniques of group observation (see "Conducting the Assessment"). Develop handouts describing how to use these techniques in more detail, and try to arrange opportunities to discuss these observations. Also include dis-

cussion of how to record observations and provide opportunities to practice and critique.

4. Gain access to the group. Obtain permission to attend group meetings. Explain as much as you can about your purpose in observing the group without undermining what you are trying to accomplish. You want to be honest about your intentions and do not want to deceive them about your activities. Tell them what organization is conducting the assessment and how the data will be used. Assure the group members that the data will be kept confidential. In some cases it may be best to have the group members sign a statement of permission to participate in your process.

Conducting the Assessment

1. Be as inconspicuous as possible, but try to position yourself so that you can observe the group members, since facial gestures are an important part of group observation. If your role is strictly to observe, you may be able to sit off to the side; but if you are going to participate in a limited way, you will need to be more a part of the group.

2. Limit recording of data during the meeting as much as possible. One of the best ways to record data is to take limited notes during the meeting by using a small note pad to jot down key phrases and impressions you want to be sure to remember. Keep the note-taking as inconspicuous as possible. If the group members see you writing down every word they say, they may not feel as free to share what they really have in mind.

3. Using the notes taken during the meeting as a guide, develop extensive descriptions of the meeting as soon as possible after the meeting. If you have been able to focus your observation on some key issues, describe what happened which is relevant to these issues. If your observation is not as focused then you will have to describe the meeting in greater detail. These field notes can be generated in several ways. The best and quickest way is to develop them using a word processor, or a capable typist. Notes also can be dictated for later transcription. (Remember, though, that this dictation will increase the cost of your observations, since someone will have to transcribe them later.) If at all possible, develop these field notes right after the meeting. Even with no notes available, you will be surprised how much you recall from the meeting and how extensive your eventual field notes will be.

4. Critique your observations between group meetings. The day after the meeting, take time to reread your field notes and reflect on what you have observed. Ask yourself what you are learning and whether you are observing the right things. This self-critique will help you be more focused for the next meeting. If you started participant observation without a real specific focus, you should find that you can become

more focused with each meeting observed. If more than one person is observing groups, it may be helpful to have them periodically meet to share notes. What one person is observing may be confirmed by another observer's experience. Also, it may assist the other observer to have a better idea of what to look for at the next group meeting.

Using the Results

Analyzing the data from participant observations is similar to the method used for interviews. If you have specific questions in mind that you want answered from the assessment, organize your findings around these major questions. If you do not have specific questions in mind, look for categories and then group the categories into themes. This latter approach is a more inductive process.

Trends emanating from the participant observation process can be aligned with the prioritized needs evolving from other needs assessment strategies. This additional information is incorporated into the decision-making process so that the next steps can be established. The decision-making process can be as straightforward as initiating planning committee discussions regarding what the prioritized needs are, and then reviewing the pros and cons of the objectives and methods to address the needs.

ELECTRONIC CONFERENCING

Reviewing the Strategy

As an alternative to face-to-face needs assessment meetings, electronic media can provide an expedient framework. Examples include video, audio, and computer teleconferencing. Equipment for these processes can be located in public facilities (such as a county courthouse), as well as in corporations.

Video teleconferencing has been slow to develop its potential for a number of reasons, including the equipment and transmission expense, and the discomfort experienced by many due to the studio atmosphere (Johansen et al., 1979, pp. 5-8).

Audio teleconferencing, while more accessible and available than video, can suffer from inappropriate accoustical conditions and a diminished ability to control the order in which one speaks (the usual visual cues are not present). Overall, audio teleconferencing uses less sophisticated equipment than the video format and costs less, but it does require more discipline on the part of the participant in order to pay close attention to who is speaking and what others are saying (Johansen et al., 1979, pp. 12-15).

Computer teleconferencing typically incorporates a grouping of experts from diverse regions of the country. Using the computer as an interface, these experts are able to meet conveniently while remaining connected with their usual sources of information. Using electronic mail, it is quite possible to transmit messages at different times and have them recorded at a message center. This enables others to review the message and respond immediately, or seek additional resources prior to drafting and transmitting a response (Johansen et al., 1979, pp. 8-12).

The advantages of electronic conferencing are:

1. It is a way to bring together people who are widely scattered geographically at relatively low cost.
2. It is a way to bring together very busy people and have them interact with one another. Using computer conferencing techniques, it is not even necessary for everyone to be present at the same time to have this interaction.
3. Electronic conferencing can be conducted relatively quickly. The typical length of a video or audio conference is shorter than the length of a comparable face-to-face meeting.
4. With computer teleconferencing, individuals are not influenced by socioeconomic status differences, which tends to occur in face-to-face communications (Rice and Love, 1987).

The disadvantages of electronic conferencing are:

1. The interaction is limited. Computer conferencing does not allow for any kind of voice or facial interaction; the interaction must be strictly in a written form. Audio conferencing offers voice interaction, but no opportunity for facial interaction. Video conferencing does offer the opportunity of voice and facial interactions, but it is more limited than during a face-to-face meeting.
2. Electronic conferencing requires participants who are comfortable with verbal forms of expression, and who are comfortable with the equipment. They also need to be comfortable expressing themselves verbally in relative isolation, without having the opportunity to observe the expressions and encouragement from other people.
3. Electronic conferencing requires access to appropriate technology. Using a telephone to conduct a conference call would be possible for most participants, but the number of people who have access to video conferencing or computer conferencing equipment is still quite limited.
4. Electronic conferencing is costly. A video conference is quite expensive; the cost for people to travel to convene in one location may still be less than the cost of conducting a video conference. An audio conference requires long distance telephone charges. If a number of people are on the line, these charges can mount up quickly, depending on the number of branch lines necessary to connect everyone.

Preparing For The Assessment

As with any needs assessment strategy, there are general steps necessary to prepare for the assessment. You need to select the participants, and develop the issues on which to focus. There are also some specific steps that are unique to preparation for electronic conferencing.

1. Select one or more major questions to consider during the conference. Since several people will be involved in this conference, you will not be able to ask as many questions as you would, for example, in a telephone survey. You will need to allow time for everyone to respond to your questions, and time for the participants to respond to each other if desired. People you involve in an electronic conference may be busy people, so you want to use the hour you have to best advantage.
2. Schedule the conference. Pick the time convenient for most people. If you are using a video network or a dedicated audio network, you also will have to consider the time available to you on the network. The relatively simple telephone conference call gives you the most flexibility in scheduling, as does a computer conference. (Remember for a computer conference, you will need to specify the time frame during which people must respond to your information.)
3. Send the participants information in advance of the conference. Remind them of the time and date of the conference, who will be included, and what you hope to accomplish. If possible, list the questions you plan to ask, so that participants can be thinking about how to respond.

Conducting The Assessment

1. Use the first few minutes for warm-up. Start the conference on time, but do not plunge into the first question. First introduce yourself and restate the purpose of the conference. Conduct a roll call of everyone who is to be involved in the conference to assure that everyone is on the line; also, this roll call gives each person the opportunity to become comfortable with the equipment and to make sure it is operating correctly and the volume is at the right level. It is a much different experience to sit by oneself in a room and participate in a meeting using this more limited medium.
2. Ask your questions in a structured fashion. One way is to ask a question, and then proceed by name in order of each person. Actually call on them by name for their response. This approach allows the opportunity for each person to respond. A structured approach is important for electronic conferencing because you may not have the opportunity to observe the various facial clues to determine who is ready to respond. It is more difficult to interject comments during an electronic conference than during a face-to-face meeting. As a result, it can be

difficult for less spontaneous people to make their comments if they are not asked directly for them.

After everyone has had an opportunity to respond, pause and ask if anyone has anything else to add before moving on to the next question. If possible, try to summarize what the group has said before moving on to the next question. For a group that is small and/or is relatively comfortable with each other, it may not be necessary to be as structured. It may be possible to throw the question open to the group and let the participants respond. Before moving on to another question, though, be sure to ask those who have not responded if they have anything to add.

3. Record the information. If at all possible, try to have someone present to take extensive notes during the conference. This person should be someone other than the coordinator of the conference, so the coordinator is free to concentrate on the mechanics of running the conference. Tape or video recording may be possible when the issues being addressed are not overly sensitive and when the audience initially can be clearly informed of its use.

Using The Results

As soon after the conference as possible, summarize the information gathered. Since the conference has been conducted in a structured manner, it should be easier to summarize the findings than for a community forum. If possible, send the summary of the conference to the participants. Ask them to review it for accuracy and send you any corrections needed. Share the information with your planning committee.

REVIEWING AN EXAMPLE

The community forum process was one of five distinct strategies employed by the Institute on Man and Science in Renselaeville, New York, in attempting to access the health concerns and health education needs of three rural counties (Hanson et al., 1983). Through the efforts of a project team, residents of municipalities within a 20-mile radius of the Institute were encouraged to attend the community forum. The team attempted to make it very clear to those contacted that this participation would be important in developing a need-related profile of the three counties.

Major steps in the process involved a keynote presentation addressing self-care for health enhancement, with a major focus on self-responsibility, followed by small group activities. In the small group sessions, participants were asked to discuss (1) their impressions of how others in the community would react to the message of self-responsibility; (2) health information, skills, and service needs in the community; (3)

barriers to health programming; (4) possible health-related projects which could be initiated, and their feasibility; and (5) their evaluation of the process.

The project team noted that the community forum, particularly in concert with key informant procedures conducted earlier, enhanced the health needs data collection process. It was noted that the community opinions offered through this process were potentially more biased due to participant self-selection. Nonetheless, the process did provide a rich resource of program ideas and enthusiastic participants.

Part IV

Self-Directed Assessments

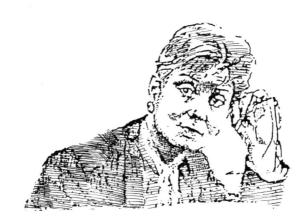

Self-Directed Asssessments are personal review procedures. Proper explanation and instruction are usually available to the general public through public and voluntary agencies. The self-directed assessments usually address primary prevention issues, such as the assessment of risk factors in one's lifestyle pattern, or the secondary prevention issue of the early detection of a disease symptom. Some of the assessment strategies combine the two aspects of prevention so that risk factors and symptoms can be detected; others expand into the additional assessment of positive factors in one's lifestyle, becoming more wellness oriented (e.g., assessing positive exercise and dietary patterns). Although some of the assessment procedures, such as the Breast Self-Examination, require initial instruction, others usually do not (General Health Status Inventory, for example). Some of the assessment inventories are computer analyzed; others are self-scored. In Chapters 9 and 10, we will review this grouping of personalized assessment procedures.

9

Self-Directed Assessment Inventories

INTRODUCTION

Individual concern for heightened levels of wellness and a willingness to take personal responsibility for certain lifestyle changes have been the recent focus on health promotion in our society. Though there is great variance in the degree of individual commitment and follow-through, it is clear that a rather potent health consciousness has arisen in our society. Recently, there have been numerous efforts designed to kindle a personal concern about health and overall well being. Notable among these was the 1979 Surgeon General's report, *Healthy People* (1979), on Health Promotion and Disease Prevention. It clarified the risks to good health, to include those lifestyle aspects over which an individual has a good deal of control: for example, smoking, alcohol misuse and abuse, poor diet, lack of regular exercise, and stress. The report called for more attention to be given to multiple levels of responsibility involving individuals, families, health professionals, health institutions, schools, business and labor, communities, and government. Particular attention was centered on the individual's role of day-to-day decisions.

The focus in this chapter is health promotion assessment inventories which can be used with individuals, to be potentially followed up with intervention, planned change, or strategies and their reinforcement (Gilmore, 1979). Some of the available formats provide a brief assessment of several health promotional dimensions, General Health Status Inventories (GHSI's). The basic intent of these formats is to quickly sensitize an individual to risk factor considerations, typically through self-scoring and interpretation. More in-depth risk factor assessments are available through Health Risk Appraisals (HRA's), which are usually longer and computer-scored. Both of these formats tend to address risk factors, or disease/death/disability inducers, almost entirely. A third type of format is provided by Wellness Inventories (WI's) in which risk factors and protective factors, or health-related inducers, are assessed.

The groundings for these types of assessments are described in a brief historical sketch by Hall and Zwemer (1979, pp. 1-3). They cite the landmark efforts by Dr. Lewis Robbins who, while serving as Chief of the U.S. Public Health Service Cancer Control Program, fostered the development of a preventive approach which would identify and appraise disease precursors, eventually leading to risk reduction efforts. In 1959, 25 health risk appraisals were completed at the Department of Preventive Medicine at the Temple University School of Medicine, incorporating the probability tables (chances of dying) which had been developed by Harvey Geller, then a statistician with the Cancer Control Program. By 1962, the term "Prospective Medicine" had been coined.

These events eventually led to a series of key events: the publication of *How to Practice Prospective Medicine*, in 1970 by Robbins and Hall; early use of prospective medicine in Canada, starting in 1971; the incorporation of the Society of Prospective Medicine, in 1974; a collaborative agreement between the U.S. Centers for Disease Control (CDC) and Health and Welfare Canada for further Health Risk Appraisal research and development, in 1978; in 1983, the first CDC Health Risk appraisal (HRA) Users Conference to stimulate the use of the process and to share information; and in 1987, in Atlanta, the introduction of a reformulated version of the adult HRA.

REVIEWING AND SELECTING A STRATEGY

General Health Status Inventories (GHSI's)

One simple process for health promotional assessment involves self-scored general health appraisals. These are usually brief, self-reported, hand scored inventories which address a few health promotion categories, such as cigarette smoking, alcohol and drug use, diet and fitness, stress management, and safety. Using very few questions or statements in each category, the purpose of this process is one of preliminary sensitization to selected risk factors (RF's) and protective factors (PF's). This process is helpful to quickly direct the attention of an individual or group toward prevention and promotion issues, to be followed up with an educational message and possibly certain health promotional activities. If the individual or group is to be involved in additional sessions, more advanced assessment procedures, such as those described below, could be employed.

Examples of GHSI's include "Healthstyle," developed by the U.S. Department of Health and Human Services; "Risko," developed by the American Heart Association; a sample of an inventory for the early detection of cancer, which is in development by the American Cancer Society; and "Operation Lifestyle" and "Eval-U-life," developed by the Canadian Ministry of Health (see Appendix A). Additional types of self-scored GHSI's are listed in Appendix D.

Computer-Analyzed Health Risk Appraisals

A more in-depth analysis of health risks is provided by computer-analyzed Health Risk Appraisals. This appraisal format typically relies on participant self-reported information related to demographics; use of tobacco, alcohol, and other drugs; use of seat belts; involvement in physical activity; use of disease screening activities (for example, a Pap smear); hazardous practices (such as hitch-hiking); and a brief health history.

The original Health Risk Appraisals, offered through the National Centers for Disease Control (CDC), were based upon an actuarial model incorporating national mortality statistics related to age, gender, and race (white or non-white). The printout from this format provided individualized information about one's chances of dying from each of 12 ranked causes of death per 100,000 population, within the next 10 years. A summary of these data then yielded an appraised health age (an estimate of how healthy one is in comparison to others of the same race, age and gender), and an achievable age (an estimate of how healthy one could be if recommended lifestyle changes are made). As an example, if a 45-year-old Caucasian man is informed that his appraised health age is 49 years, the risk factors in his lifestyle align him with the death statistics of Caucasian men aged four years older. If he will alter some of these risk factors, he can approach an achieved health age of 45 years. The printout provides information about recommended lifestyle changes based on the risk factors, as well as an expanded review of each possible cause of death and related risk categories. (Some commercial ventures garnish the basic information with charts and graphs for greater visual impact, along with more detailed explanations of the meaning of the calculations.) A compendium of available HRA's is published by the Office of Disease Prevention and Health Promotion (*Healthfinder: Health Risk Appraisals*, 1987).

The reliability (self-reported data consistency) of the HRA was examined in a controlled clinical trial by Sacks et al. (1980). The authors seriously questioned the reliability of the HRA due to certain inconsistencies in the subjects' test/re-test responses. It was found that only 15% of all 207 subjects demonstrated no inconsistencies. Breslow et al. (1985, p. II-3) however, commented on these results as possibly being due to the manner in which the HRA was administered, impacting on subject motivation, rather than HRA-related properties.

In addressing the question of validity, Breslow et al. (1985) state that "one would expect the validity of responses to suffer to the degree that a person participates in a study or in an HRA program for reasons other than self-motivated selection" (p. II-3). Another type of validity relates to the accuracy of the HRA in predicting mortality. As Safer (1982) pointed out, this type of accuracy is quite variable because it is based upon the respondents' self-reported risk factors, epidemiologic data, and clinical estimates which are used to assign values to risk factors; and death certificate data, used to calculate the average probability of each cause of death. More recent research by Smith et al. (1987) examined the validity of 41 HRA's in relation to the assessment of death due to coronary heart disease, resulting in the highest validity coefficients for the logistic regression process (e.g., Geller/Gesner methodology employed in the CDC version), while the lowest validity occurred in self-administered general health status and lifestyle questionnaries. Foxman and Edington (1987) also examined predictive validity, but used actual mortality outcomes in a community sample. They found that the CDC version of the HRA was quite accurate in predicting mortality due to all causes, specifically ischemic heart disease. They conclude that "the ease of calculation and apparent accuracy of CDC/HRA suggest that it may be an appropriate method for identifying high-risk populations for health intervention" (p. 974.)

Although HRA's have been based primarily upon mortality data, efforts have taken place to provide morbidity input into the calculations along with multivariate prediction equations (Amler, 1986). As described by Amler (1987):

> risk estimation models then will be encoded as a "risk engine," a computer sub-program designed to perform a variety of generalized mathematical and interactive functions. A parallel subprogram processes risk estimates and recommendations that are not fully quantifiable with present knowledge. The completed modules will interface with more than one format of questionnaire and printout. Additional user-defined space is planned, to add risk factors of special interest for targeted populations. (p. 1)

This newer version of the CDC/HRA was unveiled at the 23rd Annual Meeting of the Society of Prospective Medicine in September of 1987 in Atlanta, Georgia (see Appendix B). Additional types of HRA's and information for ordering are cited in Appendix D.

Wellness Inventories (WI's)

Another grouping of health assessments are Wellness Inventories (WI's). These formats are typically self-reported, computer-scored inventories which address a broad spectrum of health-related factors and their impact on morbidity, mortality, and health enhancement. Here, the health-related factors can be risk factors (leading to negative impacts in a person's life), as well as protective factors (leading to positive impacts). A number of the available formats are described by Beery et al. (1986), and in *Healthfinder: Health Risk Appraisals* (1987). As with HRA's, these types of assessments need to be reviewed for reliablity (consistency) and validity, or predictive accuracy.

One example of a wellness inventory is the La Crosse Wellness Inventory (LWI), which is part of the La Crosse Wellness Project (see Appendix C). The inventory was developed as a wellness assessment format, to be included in the overall process of assessment, intervention, and reinforcement. Initiated through the efforts of a community planning committee in 1976, the LWI—along with its follow-up, intervention, and reinforcement procedures—has been researched in university and community settings. Its primary content validity was established through a national jury process; its overall reliability (internal consistency) was calculated at .87 (Gilmore et al. 1983; 1985). Additional types of WI's and information for ordering are listed in Appendix D.

The development of WI's usually follows the process of formulating questions based on literature reviews, refining the questions, validating the questions through comparisons with standards, and calculating reliability coefficients. Richardson (1986) notes that this process is more appropriate when epidemiological data are not available for diverse lifestyle factors such as frustration, adaptive stress, and depression. With WI's, the goal is to assess areas of health-related strengths and weaknesses, not in determining the length of one's life based on health practices.

PREPARING FOR THE ASSESSMENT

There are a few major considerations when preparing to use self-directed assessment inventories. First, they are not self-reliant. They can be but one part of a total program experience, one type of assessment. Other program aspects, such as intervention and reinforcement, will need attention as well (Gilmore, 1979; Hyer and Melby, 1985). Secondly, individualized explanation, interpretation, and behavioral counseling regarding the inventory results are beneficial. It is not recommended to involve participants in GHSI's without follow-up discussion, or to send HRA and WI results through the mail. Depending upon the focus of the program, time should be built in for a clarification of the meaning of the results; particularly for the HRA and WI, include discussions about individualized steps or strategies for health-related changes. Thirdly, multiple program sessions appear to enhance the impact on participants, in contrast to singular events (Gilmore, et al, 1985; Hyer and Melby, 1985). This allows time not only for the necessary inventory analyses, but also for more in-depth individualized discussions regarding the meaning of the reuslts and possible next steps.

Fourthly, these assessment inventories are not solely aligned with one professional group. Though they have their groundings in epidemiological research and physician-to-patient counseling, they have been routinely incorporated into programming by health departments, business and industry, (Abbey, 1986; Baker et al., 1986; Edington and Yen, 1986; Shy et al., 1986) insurance companies, voluntary agencies, and other private agencies (Hyer and Melby, 1985). Fifthly, HRA's can be used to make community risk assessments (as distinquished from individualized appraisal) through the calculation of the population attributable risk proportion (PARP), as presented in Appendix E (Imrey, 1986). Finally, HRA's are targeted primarily for mainstream, employed, literate adults, though other target groups serve as major reservoirs of preventable risks (Moriarty, 1986; Rowley et al., 1986). Presently, HRA's are not as well directed to minority populations as they are to the white, middle-class segment of the United States (Rowley et al., 1986). One type of HRA, the Health Risk Profile, was developed by the Milwaukee Health Department initially to address lower income populations in that City's inner city areas (see Appendix D). For teenage populations, a "Wellness Check" assessment process was developed by the Rhode Island Department of Health (Marciano, 1986). Scott and Cabral (1988) analyzed "Wellness Check" data from 11,652 public high school students in Rhode Island finding acceptance of the process by students, teachers, and health care professionals, as well as determining that the inventory had an ability to predict high risk students who were potentially susceptible to self-destructive behavior.

Various characteristics of the three inventory formats are detailed in Table 9.1. Usually, the HRA and WI formats will be more in-depth than the GHSI. Keep in mind that the basic purpose of the GHSI is to catch the attention of the program participants by making them aware of selected risk factors over which they have some control, as well as those unchangeable risk factors (heredity, for example) which could encourage modified behaviors. The usual GHSI and HRA inventory formats focus on a negative reinforcement approach of avoiding hazards. The WI formats basically focus on positive and negative reinforcers so that undesirable behaviors can be reduced, and desirable behaviors can be enhanced (Gilmore et al, 1985; Hyer and Melby, 1985; Richardson, 1986).

Considerations for the implementation of the three inventory formats are cited in Table 9.2. One very important step prior to administering the HRA and WI formats is to make certain that enough advisors are trained for the explanation, interpretation, and counseling sessions. Typ-

Table 9.1. *Characteristics of Three Assessment Inventory Formats.*

	GHSI	HRA	WI
Assessment Purpose	General Health Awareness	Risk of Dying in Next 10 years	Health Strengths and Weaknesses
Type of Reinforcement	Negative	Negative	Negative and Positive
Scoring Process	Self-Scored	Computer-Scored and Self-Scored	Computer-Scored and Self-Scored
Administration Process	One-Time Basis	Repeatable	Repeatable

ically, each advisor can work with up to 10 participants. Plan and conduct an advisor training session which includes: Have the advisors-to-be take the inventory prior to your training session so that the printouts will be available on the date of the training; during the training session, have participant and trainer introductions, and a review of the training agenda (usually two trainers can work with up to 15 advisors-to-be); present a brief history of the inventory format (15 minutes); return and discuss the inventory results just as if the advisors-to-be were program participants, during the next 45 minutes to one hour; encourage questions for 15 to 30 minutes; discuss the advisor process you would like them to follow with the program participants during the next hour; and if there is time, demonstrate the computer program which was used to analyze the inventory responses and produce a printout.

Table 9.2. *Implementation Considerations for Three Assessment Inventory Formats.*

	GHSI	HRA	WI
Preliminary Steps	Identify Target Audience Secure Site	Identify Target Audience Train Advisors Secure Site	Identify Target Audience Train Advisors Secure Site
Materials	Inventory Writing Implements	Inventory Answer Sheets Writing Implements Computer	Inventory Answer Sheets Writing Implements Computer
Administration Time	10 Minutes	20-35 Minutes	20-45 Minutes
Interpretation Time	15 Minutes	30 Minutes-1 Hour	30 Minutes-2 Hours

CONDUCTING THE ASSESSMENT

After making the various logistic arrangements for the program, you will need to have the program participants take the HRA or WI in advance of the program date if it is a singular event (the GHSI can be taken on site), or at the first session of a multiple session program. In contacting program participants in advance, a letter with inventory and answer sheet attachments can communicate: this assessment is a very special feature of the program which will take approximately 25 minutes to complete; the results will be presented at the first program session and will be confidential; the assessment is a process for understanding the impact of one's health habits, and not a diagnostic process; from this a personal health promotion strategy can be developed; the inventory should be completed as accurately as possible since more complete responses will yield a clearer picture of the impact of one's health habits; and the answer sheet and the inventory should be returned by a specific date in an enclosed self-addressed, stamped envelope.

Many of these same ideas can be presented at the first session of a multi-session program. It is particularly important to emphasize that the purpose of the assessment is to understand the impact of one's health habits, accuracy of responses is important, and the results are confidential. Participants can be informed that a follow-up session has been planned so their results can be returned, general principles discussed, specific questions answered, and preliminary plans for health enhancement can be made.

USING THE RESULTS

Because the GHSI is self-scored, program participants will be able to quickly sense if there are risk factor areas which need attention. It is very important to clarify the process for scoring and the meaning of the score totals (usually this information is printed on the inventory), and to emphasize that this is primarily designed to provide a short, general introduction into the personal meaning of risk factors and lifestyle improvement. Participants should be informed that more in-depth assessments (e.g., HRA and WI) are available, but even these are not for diagnostic purposes. Participants also should have the opportunity to discuss their results individually or in small group sessions, with trained advisors. Usually, one risk factor area can be isolated, discussed, and simple steps for health enhancement can be identified.

The HRA and WI formats necessitate a greater degree of participant and advisor involvement during the feedback session for individuals. One process for conducting this session is to start off by introducing the meaning of risk factors (those which enhance negative health-related outcomes) and protective factors (those which enhance positive health outcomes, such as a diet with appropriate fiber content). This can be followed by a history of the assessment process, and then a return of the individual printouts.

The printout for the "Healthier People" HRA in Appendix B provides a person's present risk age based on how one completed the HRA in comparison with a target risk age. The present risk age is based upon appraised risk factors which when reduced or eliminated usually yields a lower target risk age. It should be made clear to the participants that an HRA is not a diagnostic tool, and thus is not meant to take the place of health-related examinations. Participants then can be lead through the more specific information on the printout which aligns risk rates (number of deaths in the next 10 years per 1,000) with common causes of death for one's gender and age, as well as specific risk factors for reduction. This aspect of the printout enables participants to see a potential impact of their risk reduction efforts (in terms of having a higher potential of reducing the risk related to the listed common causes of death). Additionally, participants can review what their desirable weight range is, a summary of their present habits which are considered good (for a measure of positive reinforcement), a summary of specific and general risk reduction recommendations, and gender and age-specific routine preventive services. While this process for the review of the HRA printout relates to the newer version entitled, "Healthier People," those using the older versions may be interested in reviewing the interpretation directions offered in the document, *Interpretation of the Health Risk Appraisal Printout* (Centers for Disease Control, 1984).

Overall, the three major areas for printout-related discussions with the participants involve (1) making a distinction between present risk age and target risk age; (2) clarifying the alignment of specific risk factors with gender and age-related common causes of death; and (3) addressing specific next steps which can be taken for risk reduction.

Following these kinds of clarifications, participants can be encouraged to develop a personal health plan which involves changes they are able to make. One format for assisting in this process is illustrated in Figure 9.1. Here is a point at which examples of changes would be most helpful. These could come from the advisors and/or the participants themselves. Also, this may be a good point in the program to offer educational experiences dealing with general risk-reduction issues.

Figure 9.1. *My Next Health Promotion Step.*

Risk Factor to Subtract or Positive Factor to Add	How I Will Do It and When	A Person Who Will Motivate Me	Special Considerations

The WI format printouts are quite variable. However, it can be said that general feedback sessions benefit from a clarification of the purpose of the assessment process (particularly that they are not diagnostic in nature), an individual or small group interpretation about the results which personalizes them, and recommendations for steps to take for health enhancement. One WI format also includes a listing of local resources which can be tapped by the participant, a follow-up Wellness Development Process (WDP) for the determination of specific next steps to take, and established reinforcement strategies (Gilmore et al., 1985). In accomplishing this, the participant works with the individualized data from the printout by using a workbook, and advisor interaction.

Results from HRA and WI formats also can be combined and analyzed for groups (e.g., occupational clusters) and entire communities (Imrey, 1986). In doing so, composite risk values are provided for groups which enable planners, managers, and educators to estimate health needs (see Appendix E). As one example of a group analysis, data from HRA's administered to a community group may indicate a very low level of seat belt usage. The comparison of those data with vehicular accident mortality and injury data may serve to highly prioritize a seat belt education effort directed at the assessed target audience.

REVIEWING AN EXAMPLE

During the spring of 1987 in Wisconsin, a statewide program was developed for interested school health professionals (teachers, school health nurses, counselors, and administrators), to assist them in developing health promotional programming for students and professional colleagues at the school worksite. The program was sponsored by the Wisconsin State School Health Council, which cited among its objectives,

> that the program participants will personally experience the Health Risk Appraisal Process; will review ways in which the Health Risk Appraisal process can be applied in the school setting for student health promotion; and will review ways in which the Health Risk Appraisal process can be applied in the school setting for adult health promotion.

This was a one day program; thus, the HRA's were mailed to the program participants in advance, and the advisors were trained in advance. The format for the program provided an overview presentation on HRA's for students and school professionals; small group advising sessions to which the participants were assigned, with continued group discussions during the lunch hour; an afternoon session describing the results of a statewide school health promotion project which used HRA's; presentations addressing how to incorporate HRA formats in the school settings, along with discussions on resource availability at the national and state levels; and a panel discussion to respond to participant questions about the next steps to take personally and professionally.

The key ingredients in this program included the stimulation of a personal investment and awareness about HRA's by having the program participants take the HRA and discuss the meaning of the results; provision of an example which had been conducted and evaluated in another state; provision through presentation and handouts of the resource contact persons and agencies at the state and national levels; and ample opportunity throughout the program for questions and discussion. By the end of the program, each participant had developed a personal plan for health enhancement using the process detailed in Figure 9.1, as well as a preliminary strategy for next steps with students and colleagues.

10

Observational Self-Directed Assessments

INTRODUCTION

The benefits of personal observation procedures, primarily designed for the early detection of illness, are demonstrated daily. These are referred to as Observational Self-Directed Assessments (OSDA's), since an individual is encouraged to periodically observe various body regions. Several voluntary agencies provide this encouragement through their educational materials. One such agency is the American Cancer Society (ACS), which has developed a series of assessment procedures for the public as part of its secondary prevention efforts. These include the longstanding breast self-examination (BSE) for women; the testicular self-examination (TSE) for men; oral assessments for suspicious sensations, lumps, and discolorations; and a total body review for potential skin cancer lesions. This chapter will briefly review these procedures and provide recommendations for appropriate next steps.

REVIEWING AND SELECTING A STRATEGY

Personal Observation

This type of assessment encompasses a variety of physical and mental indicators which provide an individual with a sense of his or her level of well-being. These indicators include body pulse, respiration, temperature, blood pressure, fatigue level, sensory impairment (for example, headache, ringing in the ears, bloodshot eyes), physical impairment, and mental/emotional response. All of these range from a high degree of specificity and quantification (such as pulse rate) to the more general awareness of our feelings at a given moment. The intent of the personal review approach is for individuals to be involved in these types of assessment processes regularly on their own. This approach also can assist individuals in having a sense of personal responsibility for their health (Gilmore, 1979).

As shown by Vickery and Fries (1977, pp. 29-30), the physical observations can be made quite easily and can complement medical reviews. The two physicians advocate the cultivation of an informed consumer who can undertake certain body observations, and utilize specially prepared algorithms for the next steps to take. (For example, if a sunburn is experienced with accompanying dizziness or abdominal cramps, an individual is directed to a physician; otherwise home treatments are recommended for a typical sunburn). Practical examples of important observations which can be made include owning a thermometer, knowing how to shake it down, and recording the exact temperature, rather than guessing that one has a fever. In observing one's weight, Vickery and Fries (1979, p. 29) recommend knowing an individual's normal weight, and if weight changes occur, documenting how much and over what period of time. This change-related information with a timeline can provide a more accurate picture of key stimuli which encourage greater food consumption.

Early Detection Procedures:

Breast Self-Examination (BSE): Breast Self-Examination (BSE) was first advocated by the American Cancer Society (ACS) and the National Cancer Institute (NCI) 35 years ago. A positive association has been found between the use of BSE and the detection of breast cancer at a more treatable stage. For example, Foster and Costanza (1984) found in their study with 1,004 newly diagnosed invasive breast cancer patients from Vermont that BSE was associated with the greater likelihood of an individual detecting her own cancer, reduced delay from the detection of the first symptom to histologic diagnosis, an earlier clinical stage and smaller pathologic tumor size, and fewer axillary node metastases. These subjects from a statewide breast cancer registry were followed up for 92 months, and it was found at the median time of 52 months that 14% of the BSE performers, in comparison with 26% of the non-performers, had died of breast cancer (significant at the $p < 0.001$ level).

Although there continues to be debate over the degree with which the practice of BSE consistently relates to significantly improved outcomes (see, for example, O'Malley and Fletcher, 1987), it is quite possible that a good deal of the disputation relates to inadequate measures of the quality of the BSE that is practiced. Dorsay et al. (1988) addressed this quality issue through the establishment of a one and one-half hour classroom experience which focused on training 459 women to practice appropriate BSE procedures, and then testing for competence based upon their performance technique palpation completeness, and lump detection. Their results, which included one-year follow-up measurements, indicated that competent BSE procedures can be learned from a one-session class, also resulting in the increased frequency of practicing BSE.

With an estimated 135,000 new cases of breast cancer and 42,300 deaths (second only to lung cancer deaths in females) in the United States projected for 1988, the ACS recommends BSE as a monthly practice by women 20 years and older (ACS, 1988, p. 10). It is predicted that about one out of 10 women will develop breast cancer at some time during her life, and the practice of BSE in conjunction with a physical examination

102 *NEEDS ASSESSMENT STRATEGIES*

and mammography at specified age ranges[1] can potentiate its early detection (ACS, 1988, p. 10). ACS guidelines for the self-examination are presented in Figure 10.1.

Figure 10.1. *American Cancer Society Breast Self-Examination Guidelines.*

HOW TO DO BSE

These self-examination guidelines are designed to help you feel confident in doing BSE.

1. Lie down. Flatten your right breast by placing a pillow under your right shoulder. If your breasts are large, use your right hand to hold your right breast while you do the exam with your left hand.

USE FINGER PADS

2. Use the sensitive pads of the middle three fingers on your left hand. Feel for lumps using a massaging motion.

USE ADEQUATE PRESSURE

3. Press firmly enough to feel different breast textures.

IMPORTANCE OF COMPLETE COVERAGE

4. Completely feel all of the breast and chest area. Be sure to include the breast tissue that extends toward the shoulder. Allow enough time for a complete exam. Women with small breasts will need at least two minutes to examine each breast. Larger breasts will take longer.

IMPORTANCE OF CONSISTENT PATTERN

5. Use the same pattern to feel every part of the breast tissue. Choose the one easiest for you. The diagrams show the three patterns preferred by doctors and most women: the circular or clock method, the vertical strip and the wedge.

6. After you have completely examined your right breast, then examine your left breast using the same method. Compare what you have felt in one breast with the other.

7. You may also want to examine your breasts while bathing, when your skin is wet and lumps may be easier to feel.

8. You can check your breasts in a mirror looking for any change in size or contour, dimpling of the skin or spontaneous nipple discharge.

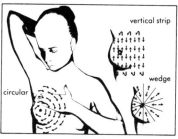

Reprinted with the permission of the American Cancer Society.

[1]ACS guidelines recommend "the monthly practice of breast self-examination (BSE) by women 20 years and older as a routine good health habit. Physical examination of the breast should be done every three years from ages 20-40 and then every year. The ACS recommends a mammogram every year for asymptomatic women age 50 and over, and a baseline mammogram between ages 35 and 39. Women 40 to 49 should have mammography every 1-2 years, depending on physical and mammographic findings" (ACS, 1988, p. 18).

Figure 10.1. *American Cancer Society Breast Self-Examination Guidelines (continued)*

BSE—WHEN? HOW OFTEN?

Your monthly BSE should be carried out when your breasts are softest and lumps are easier to feel. If you have regular menstrual cycles, you should examine your breasts at the end of your menstrual period. If you do not have menstrual periods, BSE should be done on the same day of every month.

Take the opportunity whenever you see your doctor to discuss how you do BSE and what you feel when you do your self-exam. Ask for comments to improve your BSE skills.

SEE YOUR DOCTOR IF YOU NOTICE ANY CHANGE

If you notice any changes, you should make an appointment with your doctor without delay.

EARLY DETECTION IS THE KEY— FOLLOW ACS GUIDELINES

The best means of controlling breast cancer is through early detection. You should ask your doctor where you should go to have a mammogram and how often this test should be done. Ask your doctor to examine your breasts and to check how you do BSE. By developing a partnership with your doctor, you will feel confident that you're doing all you can to help protect yourself against breast cancer.

SUMMARY: THE ACS RECOMMENDS

IF YOU ARE LESS THAN 40 YEARS OLD:

> Examine your breasts monthly
> Have a breast exam by <u>your doctor at least every three years</u>
> Have a baseline mammogram between the ages of 35 to 39

IF YOU ARE BETWEEN 40 AND 49 YEARS OLD:

> Examine your breasts monthly
> Have a breast exam by your doctor every year
> Have a mammogram every 1 to 2 years, depending on your risk

IF YOU ARE AGE 50 AND OVER:

> Examine your breasts monthly
> Have a professional breast exam every year
> Have a mammogram every year

These recommendations are intended for women who have no symptoms.

Testicular Self-Examination (TSE): Recently, emphasis has been placed on the value of males practicing Testicular Self-Examination (TSE). Though testicular cancer accounts for approximately 1% of all cancers in males, it is the most common solid tumor in the 15-to 34-year-old age group (Blesch, 1986; Frank et al., 1983). Schottenfeld et al. (1980) have shown that during the past 40 years, while the age-adjusted mortality rates have not varied, there has been almost a doubling of the age-adjusted incidence rates in U.S. caucasian populations. Worldwide, they cite that the age-adjusted incidence is highest in Denmark (during 1945 to 1970, it rose from 3.4 to 6.4 per 100,000), with high rates in North American caucasians, the United Kingdom, and Northern European countries, and the lowest rates in African black populations.

Education for TSE has been accomplished in high school settings (Luther et al., 1985) in an attempt to heighten the importance of early detection. In this instance, TSE and BSE educational modules were added to the curricula at Cleveland Public Schools, resulting in statistically significant increases in self-reported detection behavior, modest knowledge changes, and minimal attitudinal changes by the students. Teachers responded very positively to the experience. Blesch's research (1986) with 233 professional men revealed that adult males practicing TSE generally perceived it to be beneficial and easy to perform. The following process for TSE has been developed by the ACS (1982; 1986):

1. The best time to do a TSE is following a warm shower or bath, when the skin of the scrotum is moist, and the testicles are descended away from the body.
2. Examine each testicle between your thumb and fingers of both hands.
3. First, find the collecting structure in the back (the epididymis). Become familiar with how it feels and do not confuse it with a lump.
4. Then, rolling the testicle gently between the thumb and fingers, feel for lumps.
5. Testicular self-examinations should be performed once each month.

Skin Cancer Detection (SCD). Each year there are over 500,000 cases of skin cancer, of which the majority are the more highly curable basal cell and squamous cell cancers. However, approximately 27,000 of the cases are malignant melanoma, the most serious type of skin cancer, and accounts for an estimated 7,800 deaths per year (American Cancer Society, 1988, p. 13). Additionally, it has been estimated by the ACS that the incidence of melanoma is increasing at a rate of 3.4% per year. The most common risk factor is excessive exposure to the sun, with chemical exposures a distant second. The American Academy of Dermatology (AAD) has attempted to alert the public to the increasing incidence of skin cancer, and has provided a process for monthly self-examination (Figure 10.2).

Figure 10.2. *Common Sense Can Prevent Skin Cancer*

Skin cancer is the most common form of all cancers. Fortunately it is preventable and, in most cases, curable if caught in time.

"The key to treating skin cancer is early diagnosis," said G. Thomas Jansen, M.D., president of the American Academy of Dermatology. "Any unusual new growths or blemishes, or changes in existing moles or spots should be examined by a dermatologist immediately."

This year, according to the American Academy of Dermatology, more than 500,000 people will be diagnosed as having one of three main types of skin cancer: basal cell carcinoma, squamous cell carcinoma and malignant melanoma.

Basal cell carcinoma, the most common of all skin cancers, usually appears on the head, neck and chest as small, shiny, fleshy bumps that grow very slowly.

Squamous cell carcinoma is the second most common type of skin cancer and usually develops on the rim of the ear, face, lips or mouth. It appears as nodules or red, scaly patches that have sharp outlines.

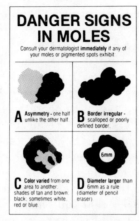

DANGER SIGNS IN MOLES

Consult your dermatologist **immediately** if any of your moles or pigmented spots exhibit

A Asymmetry - one half unlike the other half.

B Border irregular - scalloped or poorly defined border.

C Color varied from one area to another: shades of tan and brown, black, sometimes white, red or blue.

D Diameter larger than 6mm as a rule (diameter of pencil eraser).

The cure rate for basal cell and squamous cell carcinoma is 95 percent, when properly treated. Malignant melanoma, however, has a lower cure rate.

Malignant melanoma, which starts as mole-like growths that increase in size, change colors and have irregular borders, can be fatal, claiming more than 5,800 lives this year. Many fatalities can be prevented, however, by early diagnosis and treatment.

"One way to prevent skin cancer is to avoid overexposure to the sun, especially between the hours of 10 a.m. and 2 p.m. Cover up and apply a sunscreen regularly with an SPF of at least 15," said Dr. Jansen. "And establish a regular routine of monthly self-examinations of your skin. Become familiar with every mole and pigmented spot on your body," he suggested. "Any changes should be examined by your physician immediately."

To ensure that any developing lesion is caught in the early stages, a regular program of self-examination should be followed. To perform a self-examination, you'll need a full-length mirror, a hand-held mirror and good lighting to examine your skin. This step-by-step method can provide you with an early warning system against melanoma and skin cancer.

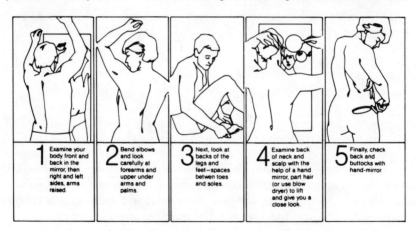

1 Examine your body front and back in the mirror, then right and left sides, arms raised.

2 Bend elbows and look carefully at forearms and upper under arms and palms.

3 Next, look at backs of the legs and feet—spaces betwen toes and soles.

4 Examine back of neck and scalp with the help of a hand mirror, part hair (or use blow dryer) to lift and give you a close look.

5 Finally, check back and buttocks with hand-mirror.

For a free brochure on skin cancer, send a self-addressed, stamped envelope to:

Sun Sense, American Academy of Dermatology, P.O. Box 1661, Evanston, IL 60204-1661

Used with the permission of the American Academy of Dermatology

Oral Review (OR). The ACS estimates there will be 30,000 new cases of oral cancer in 1988, with 9,100 deaths. The risk of oral cancer is twice as high for males, with the greatest frequency in men over the age of 40 (American Cancer Society, 1988, p. 11). Risk factors include smoking, smokeless tobacco use, and the excess use of alcohol. Realizing the recent upsurge in smokeless tobacco use, particularly by teenage males, the ACS is developing a monthly oral review process for teenagers as follows:

Check the following monthly:
1. *Face and Neck:* Are both sides the same shape? Are there any lumps?
2. *Lips, Cheeks, and Gums:* Pull down the lip. Are there any sores or color changes? Check the cheeks. Are there any bumps or sores?
3. *Mouth:* Place the tip of your tongue on the roof of your mouth. Are there any sores, bumps or swelling?
   Place your finger on the floor of your mouth. Are there any sores, bumps or swelling?
   Check around your teeth for any sores, bumps or swelling.
4. *Roof of Mouth:* Tilt back your head and open mouth. Are there any color changes or swelling?
5. *Tongue:* Use gauze to pull your tongue to each side. Are there any color changes or bumps?

PREPARING FOR THE ASSESSMENT

While it is possible for consumers to contact the agencies offering the OSDA literature and request a copy for personal use, these materials usually are offered in conjunction with a program. While dissemination based upon individual request distributes the information to a wider audience more quickly, there is less of an opportunity for clarification of the process, demonstration (many times with models), discussion of questions, group brainstorming about how the process can be personally incorporated, and the motivational aspects which a program can offer. We recommend that whenever possible a program opportunity be organized.

It is important to remind those using these materials that they are not intended to take the place of regularly scheduled examinations or other planned health care visitations; these materials are being offered in partnership with the health care practitioner in the hope that if a particular symptom[2] is recognized by the participant, he or she will seek follow-up assessments by the appropriate practitioner.

---

[2]The term "symptom" is used to denote abnormalities which are detected by the participant, as distinguished from "signs" which are usually detected by the health care practitioner. (Hall and Zwemer, 1979, pp. 21-23).

CONDUCTING THE ASSESSMENT

These personal assessments can easily be built into one's lifestyle. They are meant to be quite simple procedures, typically conducted on a monthly basis. For example, BSE and TSE can be conducted monthly following a shower, at the end or beginning of each month. Skin cancer and oral reviews also can be accomplished at those times, or they can be conducted following a routine brushing. The key to any of these procedures is practicing them at a similar time through the year so that a habit is more likely to be formed.

Though health care practitioners can offer patients individualized training in the use of these early detection procedures, time constraints may impede doing this in a routine and in-depth fashion. Group educational activities appear to work quite well in training participants with the basic assessment procedures, as well as providing opportunities for group discussion (particularly so that other questions, concerns, and vantage points can be heard), resource review, and practice with models when appropriate. The use of models with BSE training has been particularly effective in enabling participants to practice the proper palpatation process. It is also possible for appropriately trained non-health care professionals to offer delimited educational experiences to certain target groups (usually with the planning assistance of health care practitioners). Luther et al. (1985) researched the rather positive impact school teachers had on high school students following their involvement in BSE or TSE educational sessions. In each of these kinds of educational efforts, program planners should make certain to infuse information regarding the specific age-related guidelines as formulated by appropriate professional organizations (refer to footnote 1 and the example at the end of the chapter).

USING THE RESULTS

The key to an effective OSDA early detection procedure is having the participant follow up on a particular symptom or series of symptoms. A person should be encouraged to do this for a variety of reasons: (1) with early detection, treatment of disorders such as cancer is usually more successful (ACS, 1988, pp. 9-14); (2) one can obtain a more complete understanding of the meaning of the symptom from the health care professional (rather than, for example, remaining in fear of what it "might" mean); and (3) one can have a sense of being an active participant in his or her health, addressing the health promotion dimension of self-responsibility (Working Group on Concepts and Principles of Health Promotion, 1987, p. 654). By the same token, in those instances when no symptoms are detected through the use of these assessment procedures, individuals should be encouraged to view them as positive health-related indicators. In this sense, they can provide some positive reinforcement to the individual, obviously without supplanting the need for routine health-related examinations.

REVIEWING AN EXAMPLE

In 1987 and 1988 a "Breast Cancer Detection Awareness Project" was implemented by the Wisconsin Division of the American Cancer Society (Richards and Inhorn, 1988). Medical centers throughout the state of Wisconsin were contacted and offered the opportunity to provide a special breast cancer detection service to their clientele: A screening and educational program which would offer a mammography, breast physical examination, and training in BSE for $50.00 or less. The target audience was asymptomatic women 35 years of age and older who were not pregnant, breastfeeding, nor having had a mammogram in the past year. In both years, approximately 100 medical centers in Wisconsin participated, with approximately 19,000 women being screened and educated. During the 1988 program, an increased effort was made to train BSE instructors, who in turn would train community volunteers. Then, it was the responsibility of these volunteers to reach women in the community and to encourage their involvement in practicing monthly BSE.

Data from the 1987 effort revealed (after conducting the three procedures of mammography, breast physical examination, and BSE) abnormal findings in approximately 13% of the participants, of which 74 individuals had carcinoma. Sixty-six percent of the participants responded to a questionnaire which was offered and of those respondents 23% had never been taught BSE and 21% had never examined their own breasts. These results from the 1987 effort led to an even greater emphasis being placed on BSE education for the state in 1988.

Part V

Case Studies and a Computer Simulation

The following case studies are drawn from actual occurrences in four very different settings: a voluntary agency, a public health department, a non-profit community agency, and a corporate setting. These studies provide more detailed examples of needs assessment applications and strategy combinations. In addition to the case studies, a description is provided of a special computer simulation which approximates the steps one might take in conducting a community needs assessment. This simulation provides a self-paced learning activity for practitioners and students. (At the time of publication, the simulation was still in its developmental stages, but the basic format will remain unaltered.)

In addressing the case studies, here are some review considerations:

1. After reading the studies, select one case to thoroughly study.
2. Consider how closely the described situation and/or setting aligns with your present or projected professional responsibilities.
3. Note the particular needs assessment strategy which was used in each instance. Review its appropriateness for the defined target audience. Discuss the pros and cons with a colleague.
4. Determine if there are aspects of the case study which can be

beneficial to you in your professional responsibilities. What changes would you make?

5. Write down the next steps you could take in order to assess the needs of a specific target audience, or in order to support the needs assessment efforts of colleagues.

Case Study Description:
Continuing Oncology Nursing Education Needs

American Cancer Society, Wisconsin Division, Inc.
Nursing Education Subcommittee
Prepared by: Claudia Bannon*

I.   AGENCY OVERVIEW:

The American Cancer Society, Wisconsin Division, Inc. Nursing Education Subcommittee provides consultation on nursing issues, nursing education and programming to the Division Professional Education Committee. The subcommittee provides learning experiences in oncology nursing to personnel at all levels of nursing practice. Membership of the subcommittee numbers eight to 15 volunteers which are reappointed annually. Recruitment for these volunteers consists of nurses from institutions, education and community nursing.

II.   TARGET GROUPS AND AGENCY PERSONNEL INVOLVED:

Functions of the subcommittee include annually assessing the need for continuing oncology nursing education in the Wisconsin Division, assisting in the planning of local educational programs and offering courses based on needs assessment. An effort is made to identify the educational needs of the nurse generalist caring for persons with a diagnosis of cancer.

The focus group technique was chosen as an alternative information gathering process because of the inherent cost of the traditional survey method. Nurses were viewed as a homogeneous group and appropriate for focus group interactions, yielding information, qualitative in nature, with in-depth insights. Focus groups could be repeated in various geographical locations, similar in structure. The focus group technique was felt to be a useful means for developing new programming ideas and de-

*Former Director of Patient Services and Rehabilitation/Professional Education, Wisconsin Division, Inc., American Cancer Society. Presently, Assistant Director of Rehabilitation, American Cancer Society, Inc., Atlanta, Georgia.

tecting problems within existing services. The Nursing Education Sub-committee identified three objectives in developing this project:

1. Ascertain specific needs to be addressed in future educational programming.
2. Determine how existing American Cancer Society programs could be more effectively marketed.
3. Increase the awareness of the American Cancer Society services and resources.

In early August (1984), Claudia Bannon, Assistant Director of Professional Education, and Barbara Sonnen, R.N., member of the Nursing Education Subcommittee, discussed the proposal to use a focus group approach to assess the learning needs of nurses with the Subcommittee membership. It was decided that the priority should be nurses who work in hospitals, and who are generalists. There would be two groups of eight to 10 registered nurses each: one group representing staff nurses, and one representing administrative nurses. These groups would be repeated in three locations around Wisconsin. This sample constituted 10% of the targeted audience in these geographical areas, which represents one-fourth of the estimated Wisconsin Division nursing population. Julie Griffie, R.N. was asked to serve as the contact person for each hospital. The hospitals asked to participate in one geographical area, the number of their beds, the number of staff nurses and administrators invited to intend were:

Hospital	Beds	Staff Nurses	Admin. Nurses
Oconomowoc Memorial	156	2	2
Elmbrook Memorial	166	2	2–3
Menomonee Falls Community	208	3	2–3
Waukesha Memorial	405	3	3
		10	9–11

III. NEEDS ASSESSMENT PROCESS:

In mid-September, the first of a series of three focus groups took place. So that the focus group leader would not have a bias to a particular point of view, subcommittee members were not asked to serve as leaders. Judy Schmude, Ph.D. from Kenosha Memorial Hospital and Donna Pauley, A.C.S.W. from Elmbrook Memorial Hospital were asked to serve as focus group leaders. The sessions were tape recorded and the formal organized report would include verbatum quotes. The nurses invited to attend the meeting received a copy of the following discussion statement:

"We brought you here today to discuss educational efforts for registered nurses in caring for persons with a diagnosis of cancer. What comments do you have to make about this?"

In order not to pre-set their remarks, the nurses did not receive much other information prior to the discussion (or during it). The focus group leaders introduced themselves and asked each nurse to give their name and state their hospital before beginning their comments. It was announced that the sessions would be taperecorded with a 1½ hour time limit. The packet of materials presented to the nurses included:

1. A Nursing Education Subcommittee purpose statement
2. The American Cancer Society *Facts and Figures* publication
3. The Wisconsin Division annual report
4. Professional Education Materials List for nurses
5. Wisconsin Nursing Education Calendar
6. An American Cancer Society Calling Card
7. The discussion topic

A coupon for waiver of the enrollment fee for the Spring 1985 Nursing Conference was an award presented to participating nurses at the end of the session. Each nurse was asked to sign a roster of attendance.

In January, 1985 a similar focus group was held in Appleton, Wisconsin with four hospitals participating and the third focus group was held on February 7, 1985 in Madison, Wisconsin with four hospitals participating.

Claudia Bannon, Barb Sonnen and Julie Griffie listened to the tapes of the focus group sessions separately. Evaluative summaries identified needs through recurrent themes. Differing perspectives were seen in the administrative versus staff roles, but consistent within their own subgroup.

IV. NEEDS IDENTIFIED BY THE ASSESSMENT:

1. Chemotherapy
   Certification of the Administrative Process
2. Pain Management
3. Communicating with Patients/Families/Doctors
4. Emotional Support for Nurses: How to handle feelings of guilt, blame, anger (i.e., "I should have moved faster; how do I handle the family/patients response to the diagnosis of cancer and finding the time to take care of the patient despite the staffing shortages?")

In addition to these content topics there were a number of other issues discussed and other assessments made. The staff nurses groups were not as vocal or creative in their suggestions relating to learning needs of nurses in hospitals as were administrative nurses. It was obvious that the staff nurses had difficulty separating their problems as nurses from the problems of patients and families, and they were somewhat hesitant in making the comments that were made. They were not spontaneous. The administrators, on the other hand, seemed to have a broader view and they did not mention cost of programs as a barrier to participation. The issues that the staff nurses dealt with related to their own sense of frustration and being able to provide good care for their patients. They were concerned about how to help the patient talk to the nurse, how to help the patient ask for help, helping the patients cope once they leave the hospital. The nurses expressed some guilt at the end of their day because they recognized the emotional needs of patients were not being met. Resources for patients after they leave the hospital was another issue. The staff nurses' discussion had a theme of helplessness. Comments of the "politics of the system" were heard. Occasional positive ideas offered during the discussion were helpful at the local level. A local network of support seemed to have evolved in the sessions. The groups realized that within each session they had a great deal of expertise on many of their expressed concerns. It was noted that nurses in community settings are confronted with new technologies before they are educated about them.

Another issue discussed at length was access to educational programs. Administrators indicated that the distance and time was not necessarily a problem, that their willingness to send people to an education program depended on the topic and the need of the institution at the time.

The nurses in all of the focus group sessions expressed their continuing commitment to the care of the cancer patient and helped identify problem areas in maintaining quality care in our changing health care system. A letter from the chairman of the Nursing Education Subcommittee was sent to each participating hospital thanking them for allowing their nurses to participate and summarizing the information that had been gathered. Two reports were submitted to each hospital: one from the groups represented by their institution, and a final survey report from the three pairs of focus groups.

V. HOW THE NEEDS INFORMATION WAS UTILIZED:

On June 3, 1985 the Nursing Education Subcommittee met to discuss follow-up from the needs assessment. It was noted that many resources are accessible but not utilized by staff nurses.

1. The Oncology Nursing Society has developed and published guidelines and recommendations for nursing education and practice regarding chemotherapy.
2. The American Cancer Society has a catalog of free professional education materials for nurses.
3. There are toll free numbers available for the public, as well as the professional, to obtain information about cancer care issues.
4. The Wisconsin Cancer Nursing Calendar is distributed quarterly by the Wisconsin Division to all institutions with a large number of registered nurses employed. A variety of workshops on cancer nursing is offered every year in the state, and program ideas identified from the focus groups will be presented. It was determined that the nurses who participated in the focus groups will be added to the mailing lists of the calendar and future conferences.

The committee decided to meet the expressed needs by providing information to the focus group participants through a direct mail project. An ad-hoc committee was formed to determine what pieces of American Cancer Society literature should be presented. It was determined that three counties in each of the focus group session area would be included in the mailing project. It was anticipated that 6,000 nurses would be contacted. The initial mailing included a cover letter from the Nursing Education Subcommittee chairman; the publication, The American Cancer Society/A Fact Book for the Medical and Related Professions, the publication, Answering your Questions about Cancer; and a response card on which they could request a resource packet of materials from the American Cancer Society. The mailing began in December of 1985. With the initial mailing, 650 nurses returned a response card requesting the resource packet within the next six weeks. The committee discussed whether additional nurses from other areas of Wisconsin should be contacted and it was decided to mail to the 650 nurses who did respond information on the upcoming Breast Cancer Detection Awareness Project, which was a priority program for the American Cancer Society. A second mailing on the campaign, Women and Smoking, was also executed to these same 650 nurses. They have become a continued professional audience for the Nursing Education Subcommittee.

The focus group project successfully addressed the objectives and allowed development for future plans of action. Listening to the tapes has given the committee a different flavor of the learning needs than would be available from a questionnaire. This approach allows the programmer to hear the concerns of nurses, with their own emotional overtones.

It seems to be a relatively inexpensive way to obtain information.

There is evidence that the nurses appreciated being invited to participate in this activity, and that it has alerted them to the American Cancer Society and its services in a way that it could not have accomplished through a mailed questionnaire.

Case Study Description:
Child Auto Safety Restraint Project
City of Milwaukee Health Department
Division of Health Education
Prepared by: Robert J. Harris, Jr., Ph.D.*

I. AGENCY OVERVIEW

The City of Milwaukee Health Department is the official public health agency responsible for protecting and improving the community health within the city. The Department provides health screenings, immunizations, health and nutrition education, and treatment for some communicable diseases. Investigations of communicable disease outbreaks and laboratory testing and identification of disease organisms help control disease. The Health Department licenses, inspects, and enforces regulations on a variety of activities and businesses such as food, weights and measures, sanitation, animals, and the work environment to protect residents from health and safety dangers. The Department's programs are supported by the city property tax allocated by the Mayor and Common Council, plus federal and state money. Most of the services offered by the Department are provided at no cost to city residents. The 1987 Department budget was over $14 million, funding about 500 employees.

The Commissioner of Health supervises the activities of the Health Department and is responsible for making Department policies and procedures. All policies and procedures that impact on the health of Milwaukee's citizens must be approved by the Mayor and Common Council. The Commissioner is assisted by the Deputy Commissioner, Bureau Directors, and Division Supervisors. The Department is divided into five Bureaus: Administration, Public Health Nursing, Consumer Protection and Environmental Health, Community Health Services, and Laboratories.

*Supervisor, Division of Health Education, City of Milwaukee Health Department.

The Division of Health Education conducted the Child Auto Safety Restraint Project. This Division is well equipped to provide effective community-wide health education programs because of its multi-faceted approach and multi-disciplinary staff. (*See* Figure A.) The Division is comprised of five major sections: Art, Nutrition, General Program, Special Project, and Clerical. A team of 30 professional, paraprofessional, and clerical staff within these sections conducts community-wide education programs to religious, civic, and social groups in addition to public and private schools and the workplace. Most critical health subject areas are covered by these educators. The Division also conducts the largest special supplemental food program for Women, Infants, and Children (WIC) in Wisconsin serving 7,000+ mothers and infants.

II. TARGET GROUP

The population assessed prior to the implementation of the project was persons transporting children in their automobile.

III. AGENCY PERSONNEL INVOLVED

Two Public Health Educator II's conducted the assessment for the project.

IV. NEEDS ASSESSMENT PROCESS EMPLOYED

During April and May, 1980, the City of Milwaukee Health Department, Division of Health Education, conducted a survey of automobile restraint usage in the city. The survey was modeled after a national study conducted by Allen F. Williams, Ph.D., of the Insurance Institute for Highway Safety in May of 1975.

METHODOLOGY

Two health educators under the Child Auto Safety Restraint Project were trained in survey observational techniques through a slide program developed by the State of Michigan Office of Highway Safety Planning. Following this training, a survey questionnaire was developed. Nine parking lots were selected encompassing the entire city of Milwaukee, and permission to use them as survey sites was obtained. (*See* Figure B.)

The two health educators situated themselves at strategic points in the parking lots and observed vehicles as they entered. Those containing at least one passenger appearing to be less than five years of age were approached as they came to a stop. Position in vehicle and restraint usage for all passengers was noted. Drivers were asked if they were Milwaukee residents and the age and weight of all young passengers. Only city resident data were recorded.

Figure A

ORGANIZATION AND FUNCTION CHART
DIVISION OF HEALTH EDUCATION
CITY OF MILWAUKEE HEALTH DEPARTMENT

COMMISSIONER OF HEALTH

Bureau of Administration Director

Other Administrative Divisions

Other Health Department Bureaus

Division of Health Education Supervisor Assistant Supervisor

Clerical Section
Clerk-Steno III
Clerk-Steno II

Pamphlet Acquisition Inventory and Distribution

Film Acquisition

Unit Reporting

Filing and Record Maintenance

Screening Inquiries

Dictation & Typing

Library Checkout

Art Section
Health Education Artist
Commercial Artist II

Design & Layout
Exhibits
Signs Posters Forms
Photography
Audiovisual Preparation & Equipment
Inventory & Purchasing

Auxiliary Positions
Student Interns

Clinic Education
Mass Media
Text Preparation
Promotion & Public Relations
Community Contacts
Planning
Consultative Services
Committee & Board Representation
Curriculum Development
Educational Resources & Program Content

Day Care Program
1 Public H. E. II

Project LIFE
2 Nutritionists

Educational Material Development & Distribution

Program Staff
3 Public Health Educator II's
1 Nutritionist

Vertical File & Library

Rodent Control Project
1 Health Ed. Asst.

Outreach Education

Evaluation & Measurements

Door-to-Door Information & Referral

Mobile Education Van

Blood Pressures

Block Clean-Ups

High B.P. Program
1 Public H. E. II

Educational Program Presentation and Facilitation

Schools
Industry
Agencies
Community Groups

Inservice Education

Coordination Collaboration Networking

WIC
1 Nutritionist
4 Dietary Techs
1 Program Coord.
8 Clerk Typist II's

City Management Wellness Program
1 Public Health Educator II

Information & Referral

Figure B

RESULTS

The total sample included 521 children under the age of five, or 1.007% of the estimated city population (*Special Census of 1975*). Ninety-eight youths (ages 5-17) and 642 adults also were observed. (*See* Table 1.)

Of the total sample population, 66% of those in the 0-4 age range did not use any type of restraint, while the percentages for the age groups of 5-17 years and 18+ years were 99% and 98%, respectively. Regarding specific types of restraint use, only one three-year-old child used a lap belt, and none used lap and shoulder harnesses. Only 4% of the children in the 0-4 age range properly used car seats. For older individuals, only one person in the 5-17 year age range properly used a lap and shoulder harness (1%), along with only 12 people (2%) in the 18+ age group. The specific results are cited in Figures C and D.

In addition to the use of an observational survey, national, state, and local statistics were employed as part of the needs assessment. Data were obtained from the National Safety Council, Department of Transportation, City of Milwaukee Police Department, Bureau of Traffic Engineering, and the Safety Commission. Factors that were considered in this assessment were number of children under the age of five living in the

TABLE 1

Distribution of Sample by Age

Age (Years)	Number	% of City Population	% of Target Observations
< 1	76	0.8	14.6
1	102	1.1	19.6
2	135	1.3	25.9
3	119	1.1	22.8
4	89	0.8	17.1
5-17	98	0.1	—
18+	642	0.1	—

Figure C. *Child Auto Safety Restraint Project/Shopping Center Survey Results*

(NUMBERS OF CASES)

I. Do you live within the City of Milwaukee limits?   YES __x__   NO _____

II. PASSENGERS:

A. Age	0	1	2	3	4	TOTAL	5-17	18+
B. Sample size	76	102	135	119	89	521	98	642

III. RESTRAINT USE:

	0	1	2	3	4	TOTAL	5-17	18+
A. None	10	39	106	104	86	345	97	629
1. Child held by adult								
or youth	27	29	19	9	2	86	0	0
B. Lap belt								
1. Proper Use	0	0	0	1	0	1	0	1
2. Improper Use	1	1	2	1	0	5	0	0
a. too loose	0	0	0	0	0	0	0	0
b. positioned incorrectly	1	1	2	1	0	5	0	0
c. other	0	0	0	0	0	0	0	0
C. Lap & Shoulder								
1. Proper Use	0	0	0	0	0	0	1	12
2. Improper Use	0	1	0	0	0	1	0	0
a. too loose	0	0	0	0	0	0	0	0
b. positioned incorrectly	0	1	0	0	0	1	0	0
c. shoulder not used	0	0	0	0	0	0	0	0
d. other	0	0	0	0	0	0	0	0
D. Car Seat								
1. Acceptable Brand								
a. Proper Use	9	10	2	0	0	21		
b. Improper Use	19	17	5	2	0	43		
(1) belt not attached	6	2	2	1	0	11		
(2) tether not attached	1	1	2	0	0	4		
(3) improper belt use	0	1	1	0	0	2		
(4) improper harness								
use	12	14	5	1	0	30		
(5) infant seat facing								
forward	3	2	0	0	0	5		
(6) Other	1	1	0	0	0	2		
2. Non-Acceptable Brand	10	5	1	2	1	19		
a. non-car seat	10	1	1	0	0	12		
b. hookover type	0	1	0	1	0	2		
c. old 213 type	0	0	0	0	0	0		
d. other	0	3	0	1	1	5		
3. Not Used	Acceptable Brand - 16			Non-Acceptable Brand - 7				

Figure D. *Child Auto Safety Restraint Project/Shopping Center Survey Results*

(PERCENT OF CASES BY COLUMNS)

I. Do you live within the City of Milwaukee limits?   YES __X__   NO _____

II. PASSENGERS:

A. Age	0	1	2	3	4	TOTAL	5-17	18+
III. RESTRAINT USE:								
A. None	13.2	38.2	78.5	87.4	96.6	66.2	99	98
1. Child held by adult								
or youth	35.5	28.4	14.1	7.6	2.2	16.5	0	0
B. Lap belt								
1. Proper Use	0	0	0	.8	0	.2	0	.1
2. Improper Use	1.3	1.0	1.5	.8	0	1.0	0	0
a. too loose								
b. positioned incorrectly								
c. other								
C. Lap & Shoulder								
1. Proper Use	0	0	0	0	0	0	1.0	1.9
2. Improper Use	0	1.0	0	0	0	.2	0	0
a. too loose								
b. positioned incorrectly								
c. shoulder not used								
d. other								
D. Car Seat								
1. Acceptable Brand								
a. Proper Use	11.8	9.8	1.5	0	0	4.0		
b. Improper Use	25.0	16.7	3.7	1.7	0	8.3		
(1) belt not attached								
(2) tether not attached								
(3) improper belt use								
(4) improper harness								
use								
(5) infant seat facing								
forward								
(6) Other								
2. Non-Acceptable Brand	13.2	4.9	.7	1.7	1.1	3.6		
a. non-car seat								
b. hookover type								
c. old 213 type								
d. other								
3. Not Used								

city, theoretical chance of a vehicle housing a child in this age group having a traffic accident (1 in 10), number of reported injuries over a four-year period in Milwaukee according to age (1-4), severity of injuries, and injuries according to sex and age (M, F, 1-4).

V. NEEDS IDENTIFIED BY THE ASSESSMENT

The survey conducted showed that 96% of all observed children under five years of age were improperly restrained while riding in automobiles. Sixty-six percent were without any restraint. National, state, and local data pointed out the unnecessarily high morbidity and mortality occurring to children involved as passengers in automobile accidents. It was estimated that these injuries and deaths could be reduced by 91% and 78%, respectively, if children were properly restrained in automobiles.

VI. HOW THE NEEDS INFORMATION WAS UTILIZED IN PROGRAMMING

The needs that were identified by the survey and statistics strongly suggested a lack of awareness and motivation among parents to properly restrain their children in their automobiles. The Division found there was a strong need for a comprehensive education program in the city of Milwaukee to educate parents in: 1) the value of utilizing proper child restraints, 2) which restraints were safe restraints, and 3) where restraints could be bought, rented, or borrowed free of charge. In addition, a community-wide network was needed to provide ongoing education and car seat availability for those in poverty or near poverty. A proposal for a three-year intensive child auto safety restraint project was developed to be submitted to the Wisconsin Department of Transportation's Office for Highway Safety to accomplish these objectives.

Information gleaned from the needs assessment was utilized in justifying the funding of this proposal to both the DOT and the City's Common Council. Without this justification, the proposal would not have been accepted by the Common Council and the extensive existing education network and existing legislation for child restraints would have been seriously delayed in the city.

Case Study Description:
Educational Needs Assessment

Coulee Region Family Planning Center
La Crosse, Wisconsin
Prepared by: Barbara Becker* and
Susan Wabaunsee**

I. AGENCY OVERVIEW

Coulee Region Family Planning Center, Inc. (CRFPC) is a private, non-profit corporation which provides reproductive health care for a five-county area (La Crosse, Richland, Vernon, Monroe, and Crawford counties). Its purpose is to ensure and support the availability of reproductive health care, including family planning services for anyone requesting them. The services include education (contraception, pregnancy, sexually-transmitted diseases, decision-making), medical services (contraceptive methods, pregnancy testing and counseling, Pap and pelvic exams, STD screening, cervicography), counseling for sexuality concerns, relationship problems, parenting, and referrals to physicians and other local health and community agencies.

Coulee Region Family Planning Center was established in 1975. It is governed by a local board of directors. Federal funds provided 47% of the 1987 budget, with the remaining funds received through client fees and community donations.

A director heads the day-to-day operations of the clinic. An administrative assistant, fiscal manager, accounting assistant, and secretary comprise the remaining administrative staff. In addition, there is a community educator and a public relations coordinator. Medical services are provided by four nurse practitioners, one clinic nurse, five clinic assistants, and one counselor.

Services are available to anyone, with fees based on each individual's ability to pay. Eighty-five percent of the clients are at or below 150% of the poverty level. Three-fourths of all clients pay some amount based on a sliding fee scale. Services are provided five days a week at the La Crosse office, which also houses the administrative staff. There are also outreach clinics which are held at least once a week in each of the outlying counties. Staff travel as far as 75 miles to provide services to clients in these counties.

*Health Educator, Wausau Family Practice Clinic, Wausau, Wisconsin

**Director, Coulee Region Family Planning Center, La Crosse, Wisconsin

II. TARGET GROUP

The target group for this needs assessment consisted of all residents living within the five-county area served by Coulee Region Family Planning Center.

III. AGENCY PERSONNEL INVOLVED

A number of agency personnel were involved in this project throughout its development and implementation. It was begun as a project by a preceptee in community health and continued by the community educator who had the assistance of another community health preceptee. Other personnel assisted in a voluntary capacity.

IV. NEEDS ASSESSMENT PROCESS EMPLOYED

In May of 1983 Coulee Region Family Planning Center began an area educational needs assessment project in La Crosse, Monroe, Vernon, Crawford and Richland counties. The initial phase of this project began with an informal needs assessment involving five interested people who served as coordinators in each county. Each of these people convened a meeting of four to six county residents who had extensive knowledge of the county and were interested in and knowledgeable about family planning and related areas. In these meetings, which served as the pilots for this project, there were three major focuses. First, the participants identified key issues and problems related to family planning. This activity also helped in the formulation of the question for the nominal group process. Participants also suggested some possible facilitators for the nominal group process. Finally, a list of community groups to contact for the assessment was developed.

From the informal needs assessment some general ideas were gathered regarding areas of needs. People were contacted to serve as facilitators of the nominal group process. A total of 11 volunteer and staff facilitators met for two training sessions. Besides learning to be facilitators, the trainees provided valuable input into the formulation of the question used in the nominal group process.

A part-time community educator was hired in June and continued with the educational needs assessment project. She began to arrange meetings with various community groups. A total of 252 individuals, representing a variety of community groups, participated in the nominal group process. The actual total numbers of participants for each county were 77 for La Crosse, 55 for Monroe, 48 for Vernon, 42 for Richland, and 30 for Crawford. This represents an almost two-to-one ratio for the outreach counties. An attempt was made to maintain an equal ratio of males to females in the age range from 15 to 54.

V. NEEDS IDENTIFIED BY THE ASSESSMENT

Using the nominal group process, each participating group came up with a list of concerns. From this list individuals assigned values from one to 10 of concerns they thought were most important. The individual numbers for each concern were then added to derive the group value of that concern. Each concern was then carefully analyzed and combined with similar concerns listed by other groups to form categories. The values given to each concern were also combined with the values from other groups to get a total value for each category. Twenty-five different categories of needs emerged from the analysis of all the concerns listed by all the groups (Table 1). Only 12 of these categories were represented in the top five to six categories for each county. These are listed in order of priority for each county (Table 2). It is important to remember that the score value given for each category represents the total value given a specified need - not the number of people who responded. The 25 categories were then combined into eight general categories according to how the concerns could be addressed. The total values were then added to determine the priority of these general categories (Table 3).

VI. HOW THE NEEDS WERE UTILIZED IN PROGRAMMING

Because of the limitations of funding, most of the identified needs were not directly addressed. The findings have been incorporated into long-range planning and translated into yearly goals and objectives. There were two direct responses to the needs assessment. One was an increase in hours for the community educator to respond to the need for more education. Another was a more conscientious and direct approach to marketing the agency to increase the public's awareness of the scope of the services provided.

Some of the findings, such as abuse, were passed on to appropriate county agencies as need for services in that county. Involving a wide range of community groups in the nominal group process helped to establish and strengthen links with other community groups and to develop coalitions.

A task force of teachers, social service professionals, and family planning personnel was established to address pregnancy prevention in Monroe County. The task force has organized Systemized Training for Effective Parenting (STEP) programs to impact the teen pregnancy problem. Choices, a coalition of La Crosse county agencies (CRFPC, YWCA, UW-Extended Education) was created to expand options for young girls. The focus of Choices is to assist young girls with life planning. The coali-

Table 1. *Categories of 25 Perceived Needs, Ranked According to Score Value*

Need Category	LaCrosse County	Monroe County	Crawford County	Vernon County	Richland County	TOTAL
Education for Family Living	2(502)	1(445)	1(247)	8(86)	2(176)	1(1,456)
Contraceptive Education	3(303)	7(129)	5(79)	2(231)	8(60)	2(802)
Human Sexuality	1(540)	14(30)	10(15)	10(71)	4(124)	3(780)
Sex Education in Schools	6(179)	5(168)	4(134)	3(123)	3(132)	4(736)
Abuse	16(60)	4(173)	6(74)	5(118)	1(213)	5(638)
Human Sexuality-Adolescent	4(188)	2(282)	7(37)	—	9(51)	6(558)
Public Relations	11(87)	11(50)	8(29)	1(259)	5(79)	7(504)
Contraceptive Education-Adolescent	7(134)	3(190)		4(119)	12(35)	8(478)
Decision Making-Adolescent	8(114)	6(143)	3(152)	13(29)	16(25)	9(463)
Counseling/Referral Services	14(71)	12(44)	2(164)	7(91)	14(29)	10(399)
Client Education	5(186)	9(74)	11(10)	14(26)	10(45)	11(341)
Moral Issues	10(96)	—	12(8)	4(119)	7(73)	12(296)
Decision Making	9(97)	—	9(18)	6(94)	6(76)	13(285)
Teenage Pregnancy	12(85)	13(35)		9(81)	20(13)	14(214)
Availability/Accessibility	17(55)	10(59)		12(56)	11(37)	15(207)
Sex Education in Pre/Grade School	13(74)	14(30)	12(8)	—	18(18)	16(130)
Legislative Processes/Social Action	22(14)	16(12)		11(66)	15(26)	17(118)
Client Education-Adolescent	20(17)	8(87)		15(13)	—	18(117)
Qualified Sex Educators	15(70)	—		—		19(70)
Economic/Social Motivations	21(15)	17(10)		16(5)	13(34)	20(64)
Rights of Others	18(39)	15(19)	14(3)	—	—	21(61)
Abortion Laws/Funding	23(10)	—		—	17(20)	22(30)
Funding of Agency	19(25)	—		—	—	23(25)
Youth Activities	24(8)	18(8)	13(7)	—	—	24(23)
Confidentiality	25(1)	19(5)		—	19(17)	24(23)

The numbers outside the parentheses are the rankings of each need category. These were determined by the score values of each category, which are the numbers within the parentheses.

Table 2. *A Summary of the Top Five to Six Priority Needs According to County*

CRAWFORD COUNTY

1. Education for Family Living — A need to enhance family structure, communication and interaction.
2. Counseling/Referral Services — A need for more services to deal with abuse, family counseling and counseling for marital/sexual problems.
3. Decision Making-Adolescent — A need to help adolescents develop decision making skills.
4. Contraceptive Education — A need for factual material on birth control of all kinds, including natural family planning and abstinence.
5. Abuse — A need for more awareness of and education about rape, child abuse, sexual abuse, incest and alcohol and other drug abuse.

LA CROSSE COUNTY

1. Human Sexuality — A need to understand and accept one's own sexuality and that of others from a physiological, emotional, social and spiritual perspective.
2. Education for Family Living — A need to enhance family structure, communication and interaction.
3. Contraceptive Education — A need for factual material on birth control of all kinds, including natural family planning and abstinence.
4. Human Sexuality-Adolescent — A need to reach the adolescent population with human sexuality education.
5. Client Education — A need to offer medical components of human reproduction, particularly contraceptive use, in the clinic setting.
6. Sex Education in Schools — A need to incorporate sex education into school curriculum.

MONROE COUNTY

1. Education for Family Living — A need to enhance family structure, communication and interaction.
2. Human Sexuality-Adolescent — A need to reach the adolescent population with human sexuality education.
3. Contraceptive Education-Adolescent — A need to provide adolescents with factual material on birth control of all kinds, including natural family planning and abstinence.
4. Abuse — A need for more awareness of and education about rape, child abuse, sexual abuse, incest and alcohol and other drug abuse.
5. Sex Education in Schools — A need to incorporate sex education into school curriculum.

RICHLAND COUNTY

1. Abuse — A need for more awareness of and education about rape, child abuse, sexual abuse, incest, and alcohol and other drug abuse.

2. Education for Family Living	A need to enhance family structure, communication and interaction.
3. Sex Education in Schools	A need to incorporate sex education into school curriculum.
4. Human Sexuality	A need to understand and accept one's own sexuality and that of others from a physiological, emotional, social and spiritual perspective.
5. Public Relations	A need to provide more information about family planning services and improve community relationships.
6. Decision Making	A need to help develop decision making skills.

VERNON COUNTY

1. Public Relations	A need to provide more information about family planning services and improve community relationships.
2. Contraceptive Education	A need for factual material on birth control of all kinds, including natural family planning and abstinence.
3. Sex Education in Schools	A need to incorporate sex education into school curriculum.
4a. Contraceptive Education-Adolescent	A need to provide adolescents with factual material on birth control of all kinds, including natural family planning and abstinence.
4b. Moral Issues	A need to address concerns related to respect for life and Judeo-Christian standards regarding sexual behaviors.
5. Abuse	A need for more awareness of and education about rape, child abuse, sexual abuse, incest and alcohol and other drug abuse.

tion has been a part of a statewide effort in a job shadowing program, where girls "shadow" a woman who is working in a career that is of interest to them.

Coulee Region Family Planning Center also increased the presentations in the schools. Family planning staff have also been involved in helping the schools refine the Home Economics curriculum to include a course in Human Growth and Development. There also has been an increase in providing educational programs for the community, such as workshops for care providers for developmentally-disabled adults and an in-service for teachers on adolescence in the Hmong population.

Although funding constraints put limitations on responding to the needs assessment results, many of the requests received seemed to confirm the needs identified by the nominal group process.

Table 3. *Total General Needs Categories of Five-County Areas.*

I.	Community Education	4,822
	Education for Family Living	1,456
	Contraceptive Education	802
	Human Sexuality	780
	Human Sexuality-Adolescent	558
	Contraceptive Education-Adolescent	478
	Decision Making-Adolescent	463
	Decision Making	285
II.	Services	1,182
	Counseling/Referral	399
	Client Education	341
	Availability/Accessibility	207
	Client Education-Adolescent	117
	Qualified Sex Educators	70
	Funding of Agency	25
	Youth Activities	23
III.	School Sex Education	866
	Sex Education in Schools	736
	Sex Education in Pre/Grade Schools	130
IV.	Abuse	638
V.	Promotion	568
	Public Relations	504
	Economic/Social Motivations	64
VI.	Moral Issues	296
VII.	Legal Issues	232
	Legislative Processes/Social Action	118
	Rights of Others	61
	Abortion Laws/Funding	30
	Confidentiality	23
VIII.	Teenage Pregnancy	214

The numbers after each specific and general need reflect the total value of this category from all five counties.

Case Study Description:
Corporate Health Needs Assessment
Institute for Health and Fitness
Campbell Soup Company, Camden, N.J.
Prepared by: Lauve Metcalfe, M.S.*

I. ORGANIZATIONAL SETTING

The Campbell Soup Company's general office is located in Camden, New Jersey. Campbell's corporate office houses 1,500 salaried white collar employees responsible for the management, marketing, research development and support services for over 80 plants in 12 countries, totaling over 44,000 employees.

Campbell Soup Company historically has strived to play an important part in the health and well-being of its consumers. This focus on well-being is a deep-seated philosophy that has been cultivated throughout the organization and is supported by the corporate principles as stated in the 1984 annual report, which position Campbell as a "dynamic, market-oriented growth company excelling in the well-being business and committed to quality and excellence."

This corporate philosophy can be attributed to Campbell being primarily a food company, with management's realization that total well-being is a balance between good nutrition, regular exercise and positive lifestyle behaviors.

The Turnaround Health and Fitness Program is a comprehensive, preventive lifestyle management program for Campbell employees, their families and the surrounding community. The program is designed to assist in a "Turnaround" of lifestyle towards a higher level of participant well-being. It also provides the company with an effective approach to health care cost containment while offering a higher quality of life within the work environment.

Prior to the establishment of the Turnaround Program, Campbell addressed the health needs of employees and their dependents through the Department of Human Resources which oversees the medical department, safety and training division, dental offices, employee assistance program and day care facilities. Now, the company's health concerns are seen as a cooperative venture between the Turnaround Program and other departments to better serve the needs of the employees and their families.

*Director of Program Development, Institute for Health and Fitness, Campell Soup Company, Camden, New Jersey.

II. TARGET GROUP: CREATING A UNIFIED APPROACH

Both employees and management participated in the planning and needs assessment process. The process involved the initial pre-planning and development stages, implementation, and follow-up and program maintenance.

Baseline information was gathered through personal meetings and by reviewing past company medical costs to determine the current financial expenditures related to ill health and health care costs. Workman's compensation costs, lost work days due to worksite injury, medical claims, and hospitalization established a need for the organization to implement a health fitness strategy to decrease these costs. By also addressing other internal goals and objectives (for example, safety, medical, personnel), the health and fitness rationale gained additional support and visibility within the company.

Key Issues

Several key issues were important determinants in establishing an employee fitness program at Campbell.

Quality of Life. A major emphasis is placed at Campbell on quality of life within the worksite, and making it conducive to today's needs. For instance, providing child care centers, opportunities for family involvement in special events, interaction with retirees and family members are offered on a regular basis to employees.

Enhancement of Health and Fitness Levels. The company was concerned with the physiological improvements of the individual, and the development of a method to reduce risk factors that lead to degenerative disease (smoking, obesity, high blood pressure and substance abuse).

Cost Containment. Another concern was the rising costs associated with health care, worker's compensation, doctor visits, hospitalization and absenteeism. It was important to find viable alternatives the company could pursue to curtail these costs.

Human Resources. Campbell maintains a strong emphasis on company morale and loyalty. From the Human Resource perspective, the Turnaround Program was seen as a significant determinant in the recruitment and retention of valuable employees.

Philosophy and Policies. Quality of Life has remained the major priority and dominant factor in management's support of the program. The Turnaround Program is designed to offer a wide variety of health, fitness, nutrition and lifestyle choices to the employee population, their families and retirees. The Turnaround philosophy focuses on changing the behaviors and habits of the individual and offering positive support systems to reinforce change. To do this, spouses, family members and retirees have been included in the program structure.

Maximum Participation. The Turnaround Program is structured to enable all employees the opportunity to become involved. Following distribution of an employee questionnaire and needs analysis, the employee population was divided into categories that reflected their current attitude toward a health and fitness program (see Figure 1). Programs were then designed that would specifically address the needs and concerns within each segment.

The establishment of "flexible work hours" gave the employees the opportunity to choose a workout time that fit their personal work schedule. With the Turnaround Center hours of operation extending from 6:00 a.m. to 8:00 p.m., employees were able to plan their exercise at any time within this time frame provided they work a full eight-hour day.

Lifestyle Focus. Lifestyle management and enhancement is the focus of the Turnaround Program; the central component is exercise. Developing the program concept around a core of exercise has enabled the participants to have a common central focus, and offers consistent, positive reinforcement to their lifestyle change efforts. The behavior enhancement programs assist the participant who is currently exercising to develop and maintain other positive health behaviors, while offering the non-active employees a viable, non-threatening choice of health behaviors until they feel comfortable with increasing their activity level.

External Resources. Community resources, such as colleges, hospitals, health organizations, YMCAs and support groups, were identified. Once community resource information was obtained, a "preferred provider" list was developed supplying the names and services of community resources that provided quality programs and professional care. Company on-site services were arranged with special rate and class times for employees and their families at community facilities.

III. AGENCY PERSONNEL INVOLVED

Management, department heads and employees were involved in the planning of the Turnaround Program. The Director of Program Development for the Campbell Institute for Health and Fitness developed the content and strategy used to implement the program. A program manager and staff were hired to execute the programs and run the facility.

Figure 1

TO: CAMPBELL SOUP COMPANY EMPLOYEES

RE: TURNAROUND Health & Fitness Center

The Employee Health & Fitness Center is under construction with an anticipated opening date of June, 1984.

There will be a general meeting of all employees interested in joining the TURNAROUND Health & Fitness Center in April to answer questions and sign-up for the program.

ARE YOU READY FOR A TURNAROUND?
Feeling good and looking as good as you feel is what the TURNAROUND Health & Fitness Center is all about.

It means going for the TURNAROUND . . . giving equal time and attention to improving your fitness and health levels to bring the joy of "well-being" into your life and keep you in top form—both physically and mentally.

That's the TURNAROUND. And Campbell's is ready to make it happen, right here, right now!!!

The TURNAROUND Health & Fitness Center is more than a gym. It's a Well-Being Center. Once you enroll in the TURNAROUND you will be given a complete medical, physiological, and nutritional assessment. An individual exercise and nutritional program tailored to your needs will follow. The TURNAROUND Center will have an indoor walking/jogging track, aerobic activity area, and a complete strength training/cardiovascular workout area including treadmills, stationary cycles, Nautilus, Universal, and free weight equipment. Educational classes will be provided on a regular basis including:

stress management	healthy back care
time management	smoking cessation
nutrition awareness	CPR/first aid
weight management	

ARE YOU INTERESTED IN BECOMING A TURNAROUND PERSON?
If so, please fill out the following questionnaire and return it to Health/Fitness, Box 84

Name _____ Ext. _____

Dept. _____ Box # _____

Sex: Male _____   Female _____

Age: Under 20 _____   40-49 _____

        20-29 _____   50-59 _____

        30-39 _____   60 & Over _____

If flex time was implemented, what time would be best for you to use the Center? (indicate 1st, 2nd, and 3rd choices)

6am-8am _____	2pm-4:30pm _____
8am-11am _____	4:30pm-8pm _____
11am-2pm _____	Saturday 9am-1pm _____

The TURNAROUND Health & Fitness Center will provide a wide variety of aerobic, strength training, and flexibility programs for participants. Please check the types of programs you would be interested in.

strength training (Nautilus, Universal, free weights)	_____
body toning	_____
brisk walking (track)	_____
jogging (track)	_____
treadmill jogging	_____
stationary cycling	_____
aerobic classes	_____
flexibility classes	_____

Education will be an important part of your TURNAROUND. Check the programs you would be interested in signing up for (if you think a family member would be interested, please put an ✕)

PROGRAM	YOU (√)	FAMILY MEMBER (✕)
stress management	_____	_____
smoking cessation	_____	_____
CPR/first aid	_____	_____
healthy back care	_____	_____
self defense	_____	_____
time management	_____	_____
nutrition awareness	_____	_____
weight management	_____	_____
relaxation techniques	_____	_____
alcohol/drug abuses	_____	_____

Special activities involving family members will be planned. Who from your family would most likely participate?

spouse	_____	other	_____
children	_____		

What are your three favorite past time hobbies?

_____

Do you have a special talent or interest that you would like to share with other program participants? (if yes, please indicate) _____

_____

Employees will play an important role in the TURNAROUND Health & Fitness Center. Would you be interested in being a part of an Employee Health & Fitness Committee?

Yes _____ Coments _____

_____

Thank you for your time in completing this questionnaire. It is important that the TURN-AROUND Health & Fitness Center involve the employees and your input will be very helpful in the development of a quality program.

Campbell's cares about your well-being. Do you? Isn't it time for a TURNAROUND?

RETURN BY MARCH 29TH TO: Health/Fitness
                            Box 84

IV. EMPLOYEE QUESTIONNAIRE

The planning stage of the Turnaround Program was instrumental in gaining widespread acknowledgement and support within the workforce. This process took approximately one year to complete, from initial planning to opening the facility.

Determination of population needs was done by distributing a needs assessment questionnaire. This gave a general feel of the current attitudes and interests of the work site. Information on age, sex, shift, interest in commuting patterns, time most likely to participate in the program, and community resources currently using or close to provided a baseline.

V. NEEDS IDENTIFIED BY THE ASSESSMENT

The employee questionnaire revealed a very positive attitude toward developing an employee/family health and fitness program.

750 out of 1,100 questionnaires were returned. The age range of those employees who responded was between 20-67.

This questionnaire provided valuable feedback on projected times of utilization and lifestyle programs that were used to "tailor" the program to the needs of the workforce. Employees were excited about all of the programs listed on the questionnaire, with the aerobic, flexibility and weight-training classes being most popular.

It is interesting to note that the terminology used was very important in determining whether or not an employee would sign up for a class. Men selected "weight-training classes," women leaned more to "body shaping classes." Both are essentially the same program. The popular behavior enhancement classes were stress management, low-back care, self-defense, CPR and weight management. Nutrition awareness was not as popular as weight management, which reinforces the importance of choosing a title for a class that sounds interesting and appealing to the employees.

The time of center utilization that was chosen as a first preference was 11:00 a.m.-2:00 p.m., second preference was 6:00 a.m.-8:00 a.m.

All programs listed were popular with employees. (Note: only equipment and programs that could be implemented were on the list.) Strength training, treadmill walk/jogging and aerobic classes were most popular.

All educational programs offered were of interest to employees and also were checked as being of interest to a family member. Stress management, smoking cessation, CPR, self defense, nutrition awareness, weight management, low-back care, and relaxation techniques were very popular (and have been offered on a regular basis through the program).

The questionnaire offered employees an opportunity to be a part of the leadership committee. Over 100 employees responded that they would be interested to serve on such a committee.

VI. HOW THE NEEDS WERE UTILIZED

Employee Committee. An important objective in developing the Turnaround model was to provide an opportunity for indigenous leadership. Establishing an employee leadership committee was the next phase of creating ownership in the Turnaround philosophy.

The committee consisted of individuals expressing an interest in assuming responsibility for relaying program information to co-workers and volunteering for job tasks and sub-committees to coordinate the company-wide roll-out of the program. The committee consisted of 11 to 15 individuals from management, mid-management, clerical and office personnel with representation from all parts of the General Office.

The information obtained from the questionnaire was used to "fine tune" the classes offered and to schedule programs consistent with employee preferences. (See Phase V.) The lifestyle programs that were most popular were the core of the educational programs during the first year of operation.

Family members were also included in many of the lifestyle classes, which meant offering classes that were convenient with transportation needs.

Fitness Program

Phase I — Medical Screening.

The first segment of the screening is a medical evaluation performed by the medical department. An individual's personal history including any previous incidence of heart disease, high blood pressure, medical history, blood tests and other relevant medical information is discussed with the medical personnel. A three-day diet inventory is also given to individuals to complete.

Phase II — Fitness Evaluation.

Individuals not thought to be at risk are evaluated by the fitness staff utilizing the following: risk factor questionnaire, lifestyle assessment, percent of body fat, flexibility, muscular strength and a physical work capacity test for cardiovascular efficiency.

Individuals who have been determined to be high risk from their medical history and blood analysis are referred to outside medical resources for additional testing and counseling.

Phase III—Classroom Orientation

Individuals are counseled in small groups on the screening they have experienced, what parameters were tested, an explanation of the importance of understanding risk factors and how to enhance their existing health status. Materials are distributed to each participant including computerized results on individual evaluations plus information on exercise heart rates and goal-setting techniques to reinforce participation. Exercise prescriptions are then given, informing participants of the frequency, intensity and duration of their workouts, and any special concerns or questions are answered.

Phase IV—Fitness Orientation

Each individual is scheduled for an appointment to go through a workout with one of the fitness staff.

Orientation covers correct warm-up, proper use of exercise equipment, how to record their daily exercise on program cards, explanation of the aerobic, muscle strength and flexiblity components, how to monitor their exercise heart rate, and cool down procedure.

Phase V—Re-testing

Participants are tested at the start of the program, at three months, and again at six months. Results are compared with initial scores and individual programs are reassessed as needed. Examples of improvement programs are:

Exercise Classes—A variety of exercise/activity classes are offered for specific needs and interests of participants. The class schedule is flexible and adapts to seasonal changes.

Beginners Aerobics—This class is designed for the person just beginning a fitness program. Emphasis is placed on flexibility, improving muscular strength, and cardiovascular efficiency.

Jump Rope—A rope jumping class is offered regularly designed to improve coordination and cardiovascular fitness. Techniques are taught to enable participants to receive a complete aerobic workout through rope jumping.

Flexercise—This class offers valuable tips and instructions on how to stretch safely and correctly. Participants learn how to improve their flexibility and range of motion. Yoga and relaxation techniques also are incorporated.

Belly Busters—This is a popular co-ed class designed to tighten and firm up the abdominal area. Belly Busters offers specific treatment for out of shape participants.

Bunnetics—This class utilizes floor exercises and calisthenics to shape up the hips, thighs and buttocks.

AM/PM Happy Hour—Designed to improve all components of fitness, this class offers a variety of exercise techniques within its program and is scheduled for the early birds and night owl employees.

Adult Fitness—This class follows a warm-up, stretch, aerobic workout and cool down procedure, monitors heart rates and accommodates individuals who have been only mildly active on a regular basis.

Pre and Post-Partum Exercise Classes—These classes offer a safe and supervised exercise program specifically designed for pregnant and post-partum women.

Motivational Program—An important component of the Turnaround Program is the extensive motivational strategy used to maintain participation. Following the screening process, participants are encouraged to exercise three times per week. For individuals that travel frequently, a travel maintenance program is developed by a fitness technician to monitor workouts outside the center.

Inactive Policy—If a participant is absent from the center for over two weeks, the fitness staff sends a "We Miss You" card to the employee. If the participant remains absent for an additional three days, a staff member calls the participant to schedule an informal meeting to discuss the reason for the absence. This technique has been very successful and enables the participants to express concerns that may not surface without this one-on-one approach.

Monthly Awards Luncheon—A luncheon is given at the Turnaround Center on a monthly basis to recognize individuals who have improved or maintained their health and fitness levels. Three-month posttest participants are given a Campbell tee-shirt and permanent locker-room key (which can be renewed in six months if the participant remains active). Individuals are recognized in "Souper Stars," "Turnaround Team," and "Most Improved" categories. These acknowledgements are based on attendance, attitude and commitment to becoming a fitter individual, and not necessarily on skill level.

Other awards and commendations are given out at the monthly luncheon for participants who have been involved in other Turnaround programs and have met their goals.

Team 100—To qualify for Team 100, a participant logs in 100 workouts at the Turnaround Center. A large banner is displayed in the Center with signatures of participants who have made the team.

50 State Shuffle—Participants log their aerobic mileage which is plotted on a map of the United States. The trip begins in New York City (mile marker 0), winds a path through the United States and ends in Los Angeles (mile marker 3108). Accumulation of mileage is acknowledged at specific cities on the journey with a certificate of accomplishment. Once the entire shuffle has been completed, the participant is awarded a sweat suit.

Aerobucks—The Aerobuck System rewards participants with play money earned by working out at the Turnaround Center during six months of participation. Items such as sweaters, polo shirts, clocks, mugs and fitness related equipment may be purchased with the aerobucks.

Press Club—The Press Club acknowledges individuals who have met a one-repetition challenge on the Olympic Weight Bar. Tee-shirts and workout towels are earned for lifting based on the actual weight pressed with the body weight of the participant taken into account.

Participathlon—The Participathlon is a group participation challenge based on the number of participants from different departments visiting the center within a one-month period of time. Awards are given to departments with the largest percent of participation.

S.T.R.I.P.—The Spare Tire Reduction Incentive Program is a challenge between departments throughout the company to see which department can reduce the most body fat. Team members are encouraged to lose weight (no more than two pounds per week) during a six-week challenge. Tee-shirts are given to participants who achieve at least 50% of their goal loss, along with a team trophy for their efforts.

Additional Motivators—A wide variety of other incentives such as: A Battle of Department Stars, Air Dyne Challenge and recreational sports with leagues including co-ed volleyball, racquetball, running clubs and inter-community corporate fitness challenges have been used to encourage participants to maintain a regular exercise program.

Behavior Enhancement Programs—An essential element of the Turnaround concept is the behavior enhancement module. These programs address areas of lifestyle that need modification in order for the participants to achieve higher levels of well-being. The behavior enhancement programs assist in recruiting the "low-readiness" portion of the population that have not shown initial interest in the exercise-activity programs.

The classes are offered at different times during the day and are structured to best meet the needs of the participants. The most popular classes are six weeks in duration, with an hour class per week.

Turnaround to Good Nutrition—this one-hour class discusses a three-day food intake diary, recorded during the medical screening process. Participants review a computerized analysis of their eating records with a registered dietician and are given recommendations on how to improve their eating habits.

Weight-Management—This six-week course addresses the fundamentals of sound nutrition and how to realistically set weight management goals that combine good eating habits and regular exercise. A registered dietician teaches this course.

Personal Nutrition Counseling—This program offers personal one-on-one confidential counseling for individual needs. A registered dietician and nutritionist assist the individual in planning a sound and healthy nutritional strategy to encourage the development of a healthier lifestyle.

M.I.N.D. Over Weight—This course is designed to help participants achieve a greater awareness of the psychological reasons for overeating. The class focuses on understanding behavior patterns that have resulted in unhealthy eating in the past. Participants are taught how to lose weight in their present environment without dieting.

Culinary Hearts—This course offers a low-calorie, low-fat, low cholesterol approach to preparing foods that result in attractive, delicious meals. Originally developed by the New York Heart Association, the course is facilitated by a registered dietician and a food preparation specialist who combine their skills to present seminars on selecting food combinations and modifying recipes to be healthy and calorie conscious.

CPR—Cardiopulmonary Resuscitation classes are offered that combine mouth-to-mouth resuscitation and external chest compression training. Techniques to assist choking victims and other forms of emergency training are presented.

Stress Management—This course teaches participants how to effectively use stress management skills in their work and home environment. Program components include how to cope with stress, the nature of stress, sources of stress, and techniques to deal with the ill-effects of stress. Classes vary in length from half-day seminars to seven week classes (one hour per week). Turnaround staff and outside consultants are the facilitators.

Smoking Cessation—The smoking cessation program is based on a behavior modification, progressive nicotine withdrawal and maintenance format which includes additional follow-up counseling. Participants meet one hour a week for seven weeks with one follow-up session per month for three months.

Self-Defense—This course is presented using a framework of basic self-defense techniques as an effective method of self protection and viable way of maintaining physical fitness. The course integrates both neural and muscular activity and enhances coordination, balance, flexibility, power and an awareness of one's self in space. The aspect of mind, body and spirit development is encouraged and practiced. Self-defense is offered in a six-week course, two hours per week.

Lifestyle Programs—The Lifestyle Programs are designed to attract new members to the Turnaround Program and add an element of fun and variety to the structure. The programs offer a way of penetrating the office and work population by "massaging" one's attitude on adapting positive lifestyle behaviors.

Exer-Breaks—At-desk exercise breaks are offered to departments within the General Office and in the conference rooms during the customary break time of 10:00 a.m. and 2:00 p.m.

Souped Up Walks—Fitness walking groups are scheduled during the 10:00 a.m. and 2:00 p.m. break times when the weather allows. These groups are led by Turnaround staff around the General Office grounds with accompanying upbeat music.

Soup to Nuts—Table top cards are displayed in the cafeteria with information on exercise, nutrition and lifestyle. At the end of the month a quiz on the information is given. Winners receive a specially designed tee-shirt. Information changes on a monthly basis.

Kinderfit—Exercise classes are offered daily to the Campbell Day Care Center located adjacent to the Turnaround Center. Instruction is given on hand-eye coordination and the components of exercise in a fun and enjoyable manner are presented to the children.

Live It Up—This program involves a local medical center that cares for senior citizens. The Turnaround staff encourages patients to express themselves and participate in the activities that promote range of motion and flexibility. There has been success in blending the Kinderfit and Live It Up programs through "Adopt a Grandparent," and "Adopt a Grandchild" activities.

VII. COMMENTARY

To have a major lasting effect on Campbell's bottom line and to improve substantially the quality of work life, we must address the corporation in its totality, from upper level management to office worker to line worker, and develop programs that meet their respective needs.

Commitment at the start-up stage means believing in a mutually agreed upon set of quality of life values and being willing to take the risk to apply those values at the worksite. Although not a promise for perfection, a health and fitness process offers the potential for a more productive work force and higher quality of work life. Real commitment means believing in these benefits enough to be willing to live with the costs and the time required to process the change.

The very core of integrating the health and fitness process into the total employee work force fundamentally deals with the realization that a company's most valuable resource is its employees.

For corporate programs, our challenge has been how to entice participation in programs that usually are scheduled into the daily framework of office flex hours and are budgeted through medical, human resources, or other corporate services departments.

For blue collar or hourly personnel, the issues are a bit more complex. The bottom line production cost becomes the primary concern for plant management. Workers are clocked in and out, vary their shifts regularly and find working six days a week part of the job. This system, although vastly different from the climate of the corporate turf, has the potential for developing a healthy work culture if properly executed, and if the present system of operation can be revised to support positive change.

As a quality of work life process evolves, the potential for an integrated system that also offers flexible work hours, day care, employee assistance programs, nutrition education, preventive medicine, safety programs and Quality Circle opportunities becomes possible. Ultimately, we try to influence the way that the organization is perceived by the employee and enhance the quality of work generated by that employee. Through a viable quality of working life strategy developed and enhanced by continually assessing the needs of the employee population, we can actively pursue a long-term process of change toward a healthier lifestyle and work style for all.

Computer-Simulated Community Needs Assessment

Prepared by: Jay V. Schindler, Ph.D.*

INTRODUCTION

Unlike the preceding case studies, this case study describes an intervention that takes place in a simulated environment on the computer. This simulation is a learning tool for beginning community health educators to practice intervention skills on the simulated community. Users may interview key people in the community, conduct a needs assessment, plan and implement community health education programs, and receive feedback from program participants and community leaders. Unlike the real world, users can make costly mistakes without damaging any real community, can stop the simulation and start over from scratch, and can examine the underlying variables that control the mathematical manipulations of the simulation. This simulation, Community Inneede, provides enough interaction to make it challenging and enjoyable to users, yet friendly enough for beginners to try. The instructors who use Community Inneede also are able to vary the major health problems of the community, making the situations as easy or as difficult as they would like.

I. BRIEF OVERVIEW OF THE AGENCY/ORGANIZATION

Each user begins the program as a newly hired member of the county public health department. The public health department conducts the typical activities you would expect of such an agency, but has hired the user as a health educator to develop *new* programming activities that would advance the health of their target group. The director of the public health department has a few introductory comments to make to the user, but for the most part, lets the new health educator work freely. In fact,

*Associate Professor, Health Education Department, University of Wisconsin-LaCrosse.

the director states in the simulation, "I hired you because you showed initiative, as well as an ability to discover where health education programs are most needed. I will give you some feedback at the 60-day review that all new employees receive, but until then I'll let you do your own thing. Go to it!"

II. TARGET GROUP

The target group consists of a medium sized community (60,000 population) with a variety of subgroups. Although the predominant group consists of white, middle-class, blue-collar workers, there are minority groups that comprise most of the lower-class members in Community Inneede. The graphics display of the simulation shows a map of the community, and it becomes evident there are geographic localizations of the minority groups within the community. Any needs assessment will have to keep these geographic dissimilarities in mind if the needs assessment is to be considered an accurate representation of the community.

III. AGENCY PERSONNEL INVOLVED

For the Community Inneede simulation, the user is the only person actively involved in the needs assessment for health education programming efforts. This allows the simulation user to develop an understanding of the needs assessment process while deciding what activities to conduct. In the process of conducting a needs assessment, the user can request feedback from a variety of key characters in the simulation, including the director of the public health department.

IV. NEEDS ASSESSMENT PROCESSES EMPLOYED

Within the Community Inneede simulation, two major forms of needs assessment are permitted at this time: a key informant approach and a community survey approach. (The latter approach can be conducted via telephone survey, mail survey, or door-to-door interview process.)

Within the simulation is a database of answers key informants would give to answer specific questions about the community. A few examples of key informants are: the executive director of the local American Red Cross chapter, the chair of the Extended Education Services at the local community college, the pediatrician heading up the local hospital's community education services, and the Health Services coordinator at the local YMCA—YWCA. Key informants include representatives of the target group subpopulations as well as representatives of education/intervention services in the community.

The simulation is limited to a specific set of needs assessment questions from which the user must choose. Some questions yield very helpful answers, while other questions yield answers that are misleading or too vague to be of any help. The key for users is to detect the quality of the question being asked; poorly worded questions will yield mostly vague answers, while clear, direct questions can provide much insight into the community's needs.

The community survey approach is fairly simple, but does provide the user an opportunity to specify a region of the community in which the survey will take place. The user can then specify the proportion of residences to be surveyed in the region already delineated. Thus, for example, the user can specify a region of the community mostly inhabited by minority members, and can then request a survey of 30% of all residences in that region. If the user wants to, the region can equal the whole community in order to conduct a complete survey.

In order to make the simulation more realistic, every needs assessment activity has both time and monetary budget. The more extensive the user's needs assessment, the more expensive and time-consuming it will be. Cost overruns for poor data provide negative feedback to the user, while judicious needs assessments that provide quality data result in positive feedback to the user.

V. NEEDS IDENTIFIED BY THE ASSESSMENT

The Community Inneede simulation comes with a database already on the disk. The database is set up to indicate a need for smoking cessation health education programs within the blue-collar workers, and a need for teenage pregnancy education among the minority group members in the community. This database, however, can be altered by the instructor running the simulation. Using a special menu, the instructor can select the nature and extent of specific problems within the Community Inneede simulation. The instructor can make the community's specific health needs as obvious or as hidden as he or she would like, thus altering the level of difficulty associated with the needs assessment activity.

VI. HOW THE NEEDS CAN BE UTILIZED IN PROGRAMMING

If the Community Inneede simulation user correctly identified the major needs of the community, then the Intervention Stage that followed would be correctly targeted. In the Intervention Stage, the user specifies: the type of intervention (mass media campaign, educational program, screening assessment, or organizational change); the content area (exercise & fitness, nutrition and diet, stress management, cancer prevention, smoking cessation, hypertension, or sexual life education); and the type of intervention (enhance awareness, provide motivation, disseminate information, or train in skills).

VII.   ADDITIONAL COMMENTARY

Community Inneede is still in the programming stage as of this writing. Although the description of the simulation has been worked out fairly completely, the final form of the Community Inneede simulation may be different than what is described above. Many factors will influence the final format, most of all the ease of use for those doing the simulation. Anyone who would like further information on the status of the simulation should contact Dr. Jay Schindler at the University of Wisconsin-La Crosse.

Appendices

Appendix A
Examples of General Health
Status Inventories

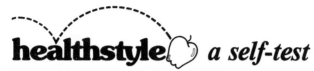

healthstyle: a self-test

All of us want good health. But many of us do not know how to be as healthy as possible. Health experts now describe *lifestyle* as one of the most important factors affecting health. In fact, it is estimated that as many as seven of the ten leading causes of death could be reduced through common-sense changes in lifestyle. That's what this brief test, developed by the Public Health Service, is all about. Its purpose is simply to tell you how well you are doing to stay healthy. The behaviors covered in the test are recommended for most Americans. Some of them may not apply to persons with certain chronic diseases or handicaps, or to pregnant women. Such persons may require special instructions from their physicians.

Almost Always / Sometimes / Almost Never

Cigarette Smoking

If you never smoke, enter a score of 10 for this section and go to the next section on *Alcohol and Drugs*.

1. I avoid smoking cigarettes. 2 1 0

2. I smoke only low tar and nicotine cigarettes *or* I smoke a pipe or cigars. 2 1 0

Smoking Score: _____

Alcohol and Drugs

1. I avoid drinking alcoholic beverages *or* I drink no more than 1 or 2 drinks a day. 4 1 0

2. I avoid using alcohol or other drugs (especially illegal drugs) as a way of handling stressful situations or the problems in my life. 2 1 0

3. I am careful not to drink alcohol when taking certain medicines (for example, medicine for sleeping, pain, colds, and allergies), or when pregnant. 2 1 0

4. I read and follow the label directions when using prescribed and over-the-counter drugs. 2 1 0

Alcohol and Drugs Score: _____

Eating Habits

1. I eat a variety of foods each day, such as fruits and vegetables, whole grain breads and cereals, lean meats, dairy products, dry peas and beans, and nuts and seeds. 4 1 0

2. I limit the amount of fat, saturated fat, and cholesterol I eat (including fat on meats, eggs, butter, cream, shortenings, and organ meats such as liver). 2 1 0

3. I limit the amount of salt I eat by cooking with only small amounts, not adding salt at the table, and avoiding salty snacks. 2 1 0

4. I avoid eating too much sugar (especially frequent snacks of sticky candy or soft drinks). 2 1 0

Eating Habits Score: _____

Exercise/Fitness

1. I maintain a desired weight, avoiding overweight and underweight. 3 1 0

2. I do vigorous exercises for 15-30 minutes at least 3 times a week (examples include running, swimming, brisk walking). 3 1 0

3. I do exercises that enhance my muscle tone for 15-30 minutes at least 3 times a week (examples include yoga and calisthenics). 2 1 0

4. I use part of my leisure time participating in individual, family, or team activities that increase my level of fitness (such as gardening, bowling, golf, and baseball). 2 1 0

Exercise/Fitness Score: _____

Stress Control

1. I have a job or do other work that I enjoy. 2 1 0

2. I find it easy to relax and express my feelings freely. 2 1 0

3. I recognize early, and prepare for, events or situations likely to be stressful for me. 2 1 0

4. I have close friends, relatives, or others whom I can talk to about personal matters and call on for help when needed. 2 1 0

5. I participate in group activities (such as church and community organizations) or hobbies that I enjoy. 2 1 0

Stress Control Score: _____

Safety

1. I wear a seat belt while riding in a car. 2 1 0

2. I avoid driving while under the influence of alcohol and other drugs. 2 1 0

3. I obey traffic rules and the speed limit when driving. 2 1 0

4. I am careful when using potentially harmful products or substances (such as household cleaners, poisons, and electrical devices). 2 1 0

5. I avoid smoking in bed. 2 1 0

Safety Score: _____

149

What Your Scores Mean to YOU

Scores of 9 and 10

Excellent! Your answers show that you are aware of the importance of this area to your health. More important, you are putting your knowledge to work for you by practicing good health habits. As long as you continue to do so, this area should not pose a serious health risk. It's likely that you are setting an example for your family and friends to follow. Since you got a very high test score on this part of the test, you may want to consider other areas where your scores indicate room for improvement.

Scores of 6 to 8

Your health practices in this area are good, but there is room for improvement. Look again at the items you answered with a "Sometimes" or "Almost Never." What changes can you make to improve your score? Even a small change can often help you achieve better health.

Scores of 3 to 5

Your health risks are showing! Would you like more information about the risks you are facing and about why it is important for you to change these behaviors. Perhaps you need help in deciding how to successfully make the changes you desire. In either case, help is available.

Scores of 0 to 2

Obviously, you were concerned enough about your health to take the test, but your answers show that you may be taking serious and unnecessary risks with your health. Perhaps you are not aware of the risks and what to do about them. You can easily get the information and help you need to improve, if you wish. The next step is up to you.

YOU Can Start Right Now!

In the test you just completed were numerous suggestions to help you reduce your risk of disease and premature death. Here are some of the most significant:

 Avoid cigarettes. Cigarette smoking is the single most important preventable cause of illness and early death. It is especially risky for pregnant women and their unborn babies. Persons who stop smoking reduce their risk of getting heart disease and cancer. So if you're a cigarette smoker, think twice about lighting that next cigarette. If you choose to continue smoking, try decreasing the number of cigarettes you smoke and switching to a low tar and nicotine brand.

 Follow sensible drinking habits. Alcohol produces changes in mood and behavior. Most people who drink are able to control their intake of alcohol and to avoid undesired, and often harmful, effects. Heavy, regular use of alcohol can lead to cirrhosis of the liver, a leading cause of death. Also, statistics clearly show that mixing drinking and driving is often the cause of fatal or crippling accidents. So if you drink, do it wisely and in moderation. *Use care in taking drugs.* Today's greater use of drugs—both legal and illegal—is one of our most serious health risks. Even some drugs prescribed by your doctor can be dangerous if taken when drinking alcohol or before driving. Excessive or continued use of tranquilizers (or

"pep pills") can cause physical and mental problems. Using or experimenting with illicit drugs such as marijuana, heroin, cocaine, and PCP may lead to a number of damaging effects or even death.

 Eat sensibly. Overweight individuals are at greater risk for diabetes, gall bladder disease, and high blood pressure. So it makes good sense to maintain proper weight. But good eating habits also mean holding down the amount of fat (especially saturated fat), cholesterol, sugar and salt in your diet. If you must snack, try nibbling on fresh fruits and vegetables. You'll feel better—and look better, too.

 Exercise regularly. Almost everyone can benefit from exercise—and there's some form of exercise almost everyone can do. (If you have any doubt, check first with your doctor.) Usually, as little as 15-30 minutes of vigorous exercise three times a week will help you have a healthier heart, eliminate excess weight, tone up sagging muscles, and sleep better. Think how much difference all these improvements could make in the way you feel!

 Learn to handle stress. Stress is a normal part of living; everyone faces it to some degree. The causes of stress can be good or bad, desirable or undesirable (such as a promotion on the job or the loss of a spouse). Properly handled, stress need not be a problem. But unhealthy responses to stress—such as driving too fast or erratically, drinking too much, or prolonged anger or grief—can cause a variety of physical and mental problems. Even on a very busy day, find a few minutes to slow down and relax. Talking over a problem with someone you trust can often help you find a satisfactory solution. Learn to distinguish between things that are "worth fighting about" and things that are less important.

 Be safety conscious. Think "safety first" at home, at work, at school, at play, and on the highway. Buckle seat belts and obey traffic rules. Keep poisons and weapons out of the reach of children, and keep emergency numbers by your telephone. When the unexpected happens, you'll be prepared.

Where Do You Go From Here:

Start by asking yourself a few frank questions: *Am I really doing all I can to be as healthy as possible? What steps can I take to feel better? Am I willing to begin now?* If you scored low in one or more *sections* of the test, decide what changes you want to make for improvement. You might pick that aspect of your lifestyle where you feel you have the best chance for success and tackle that one first. Once you have improved your score there, go on to other areas.

If you already have tried to change your health habits (to stop smoking or exercise regularly, for example), don't be discouraged if you haven't yet succeeded. The difficulty you have encountered may be due to influences you've never really thought about—such as advertising—or to a lack

of support and encouragement. Understanding these influences is an important step toward changing the way they affect you.

There's Help Available. In addition to personal actions you can take on your own, there are community programs and groups (such as the YMCA or the local chapter of the American Heart Association) that can assist you and your family to make the changes you want to make. If you want to know more about these groups or about health risks, contact your local health department or the National Health Information Clearinghouse. There's a lot you can do to stay healthy or to improve your health—and there are organizations that can help you. Start a new HEALTHSTYLE today!

For more copies of this publication, or for a catalog of other publications, contact:

Wisconsin Clearinghouse
P.O. Box 1468
Madison, Wisconsin 53701

This publication was partly funded through the Wisconsin Department of Health and Social Services.

Reprinted with the permission of the Wisconsin Clearinghouse

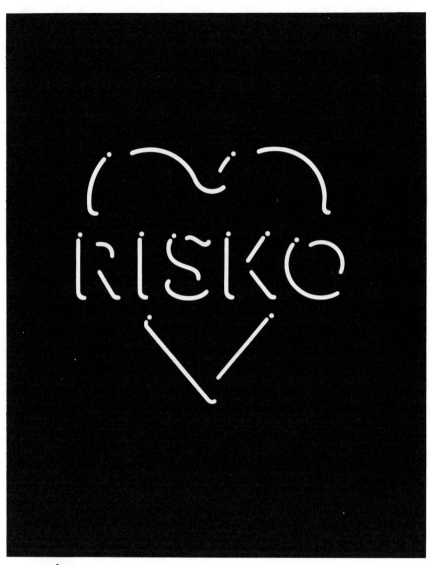

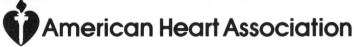
American Heart Association

Reproduced with permission. © Risko. American Heart Association.

MEN

Find the column for your age group. Everyone starts with a score of 10 points. Work down the page *adding* points to your score or *subtracting* points from your score.

	54 OR YOUNGER	55 OR OLDER
	STARTING SCORE **10**	STARTING SCORE **10**

1. WEIGHT

Locate your weight category in the table below. If you are in

		54 OR YOUNGER	55 OR OLDER
	weight category A	SUBTRACT 2	SUBTRACT 2
	weight category B	SUBTRACT 1	ADD 0
	weight category C	ADD 1	ADD 1
	weight category D	ADD 2	ADD 3
		EQUALS ☐	EQUALS ☐

2. SYSTOLIC BLOOD PRESSURE

Use the "first" or "higher" number from your most recent blood pressure measurement. If you do not know your blood pressure, estimate it by using the letter for your weight category. If your blood pressure is

		54 OR YOUNGER	55 OR OLDER
A	119 or less	SUBTRACT 1	SUBTRACT 5
B	between 120 and 139	ADD 0	SUBTRACT 2
	between 140 and 159	ADD 0	ADD 1
D	160 or greater	ADD 1	ADD 4
		EQUALS ☐	EQUALS ☐

3. BLOOD CHOLESTEROL LEVEL

Use the number from your most recent blood cholesterol test. If you do not know your blood cholesterol, estimate it by using the letter for your weight category. If your blood cholesterol is

		54 OR YOUNGER	55 OR OLDER
A	199 or less	SUBTRACT 2	SUBTRACT 1
B	between 200 and 224	SUBTRACT 1	SUBTRACT 1
	between 225 and 249	ADD 0	ADD 0
D	250 or higher	ADD 1	ADD 0
		EQUALS ☐	EQUALS ☐

4. CIGARETTE SMOKING

If you

(If you smoke a pipe, but not cigarettes, use the same score adjustment as those cigarette smokers who smoke less than a pack a day.)

		54 OR YOUNGER	55 OR OLDER
	do not smoke	SUBTRACT 1	SUBTRACT 2
	smoke less than a pack a day	ADD 0	SUBTRACT 1
	smoke a pack a day	ADD 1	ADD 0
	smoke more than a pack a day	ADD 2	ADD 3
		FINAL SCORE EQUALS ☐	FINAL SCORE EQUALS ☐

WEIGHT TABLE FOR MEN

Look for your height (without shoes) in the far left column and then read across to find the category into which your weight (in indoor clothing) would fall.

YOUR HEIGHT FT IN	WEIGHT CATEGORY (lbs.)			
	A	B		D
5 1	up to 123	124-148	149-173	174 plus
5 2	up to 126	127-152	153-178	179 plus
5 3	up to 129	130-156	157-182	183 plus
5 4	up to 132	133-160	161-186	187 plus
5 5	up to 135	136-163	164-190	191 plus
5 6	up to 139	140-168	169-196	197 plus
5 7	up to 144	145-174	175-203	204 plus
5 8	up to 148	149-179	180-209	210 plus
5 9	up to 152	153-184	185-214	215 plus
5 10	up to 157	158-190	191-221	222 plus
5 11	up to 161	162-194	195-227	228 plus
6 0	up to 165	166-199	200-232	233 plus
6 1	up to 170	171-205	206-239	240 plus
6 2	up to 175	176-211	212-246	247 plus
6 3	up to 180	181-217	218-253	254 plus
6 4	up to 185	186-223	224-260	261 plus
6 5	up to 190	191-229	230-267	268 plus
6 6	up to 195	196-235	236-274	275 plus
ESTIMATE OF SYSTOLIC BLOOD PRESSURE	119 or less			160 or more
ESTIMATE OF BLOOD CHOLESTEROL	199 or less			250 or more

Because both blood pressure and blood cholesterol are related to weight, an estimate of these risk factors for each weight category is printed at the bottom of the table.

© 1981 American Heart Association

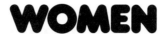
WOMEN

Find the column for your age group. Everyone starts with a score of 10 points. Work down the page *adding* points to your score or *subtracting* points from your score.

		54 OR YOUNGER	55 OR OLDER

1. WEIGHT

Locate your weight category in the table below. If you are in

		STARTING SCORE **10**	STARTING SCORE **10**
☐	weight category A	SUBTRACT 2	SUBTRACT 2
▨	weight category B	SUBTRACT 1	SUBTRACT 1
▤	weight category C	ADD 1	ADD 0
■	weight category D	ADD 2	ADD 1
		EQUALS ☐	EQUALS ☐

2. SYSTOLIC BLOOD PRESSURE

Use the "first" or "higher" number from your most recent blood pressure measurement. If you do not know your blood pressure, estimate it by using the letter for your weight category. If your blood pressure is

A	119 or less	SUBTRACT 2	SUBTRACT 3
B	between 120 and 139	SUBTRACT 1	ADD 0
	between 140 and 159	ADD 0	ADD 3
D	160 or greater	ADD 1	ADD 6
		EQUALS ☐	EQUALS ☐

3. BLOOD CHOLESTEROL LEVEL

Use the number from your most recent blood cholesterol test. If you do not know your blood cholesterol, estimate it by using the letter for your weight category. If your blood cholesterol is

A	199 or less	SUBTRACT 1	SUBTRACT 3
B	between 200 and 224	ADD 0	SUBTRACT 1
	between 225 and 249	ADD 0	ADD 1
D	250 or higher	ADD 1	ADD 3
		EQUALS ☐	EQUALS ☐

4. CIGARETTE SMOKING

If you

☐	do not smoke	SUBTRACT 1	SUBTRACT 2
	smoke less than a pack a day	ADD 0	SUBTRACT 1
	smoke a pack a day	ADD 1	ADD 1
■	smoke more than a pack a day	ADD 2	ADD 4
		EQUALS ☐	EQUALS ☐

5. ESTROGEN USE

Birth control pills and hormone drugs contain estrogen. A few examples are: ·Premarin ·Ogan ·Menstranol ·Provera ·Evex ·Menest ·Estinyl ·Meurium

· Have you ever taken estrogen for five or more years in a row?
· Are you age 35 years or older and are now taking estrogen?

☐	No to both questions	ADD 0	ADD 0
■	Yes to one or both questions	ADD 1	ADD 3

FINAL SCORE EQUALS ☐	FINAL SCORE EQUALS ☐

	YOUR HEIGHT FT IN	WEIGHT CATEGORY (lbs.)			
		A	B		D
WEIGHT TABLE FOR WOMEN Look for your height (without shoes) in the far left column and then read across to find the category into which your weight (in indoor clothing) would fall.	4 8	up to 101	102-122	123-143	144 plus	Because both blood pressure and blood cholesterol are related to weight, an estimate of these risk factors for each weight category is printed at the bottom of the table.
	4 9	up to 103	104-125	126-146	147 plus	
	4 10	up to 106	107-128	129-150	151 plus	
	4 11	up to 109	110-132	133-154	155 plus	
	5 0	up to 112	113-136	137-158	159 plus	
	5 1	up to 115	116-139	140-162	163 plus	
	5 2	up to 119	120-144	145-168	169 plus	
	5 3	up to 122	123-148	149-172	173 plus	
	5 4	up to 127	128-154	155-179	180 plus	
	5 5	up to 131	132-158	159-185	186 plus	
	5 6	up to 135	136-163	164-190	191 plus	
	5 7	up to 139	140-168	169-196	197 plus	
	5 8	up to 143	144-173	174-202	203 plus	
	5 9	up to 147	148-178	179-207	208 plus	
	5 10	up to 151	152-182	183-213	214 plus	
	5 11	up to 155	156-187	188-218	219 plus	
	6 0	up to 159	160-191	192-224	225 plus	
	6 1	up to 163	164-196	197-229	230 plus	
ESTIMATE OF SYSTOLIC BLOOD PRESSURE		119 or less			160 or more	
ESTIMATE OF BLOOD CHOLESTEROL		199 or less			250 or more	

WHAT YOUR SCORE MEANS

0-4
You have one of the lowest risks of Heart Disease for your age and sex.

5-9
You have a low to moderate risk of Heart Disease for your age and sex but there is some room for improvement.

10-14
You have a moderate to high risk of Heart Disease for your age and sex. with considerable room for improvement on some factors.

15-19
You have a high risk of developing Heart Disease for your age and sex with a great deal of room for improvement on all factors.

20 & over
You have a very high risk of developing Heart Disease for your age and sex and should take immediate action on all risk factors.

WARNING

* If you have diabetes, gout or a family history of heart disease, your actual risk will be greater than indicated by this appraisal.
* If you do not know your current blood pressure or blood cholesterol level, you should visit your physician or health center to have them measured. Then figure your score again for a more accurate determination of your risk.
* If you are overweight, have high blood pressure or high blood cholesterol, or smoke cigarettes, your long-term risk of heart disease is increased even if your risk in the next several years is low.

HOW TO REDUCE YOUR RISK

* Try to quit smoking permanently. There are many programs available.
* Have your blood pressure checked regularly, preferably every twelve months after age 40. If your blood pressure is high, see your physician. Remember blood pressure medicine is only effective if taken regularly.
* Consider your daily exercise (or lack of it). A half hour of brisk walking, swimming or other enjoyable activity should not be difficult to fit into your day.
* Give some serious thought to your diet. If you are overweight, or eat a lot of foods high in saturated fat or cholesterol (whole milk, cheese, eggs, butter, fatty foods, fried foods) then changes should be made in your diet. Look for the American Heart Association Cookbook at your local bookstore.
* Visit or write your local Heart Association for further information and copies of free pamphlets on many related subjects including:
  * Reducing your risk of heart attack.
  * Controlling high blood pressure.
  * Eating to keep your heart healthy.
  * How to stop smoking.
  * Exercising for good health.

SOME WORDS OF CAUTION

* If you have diabetes, gout, or a family history of heart disease, your real risk of developing heart disease will be greater than indicated by your RISKO score. If your score is high and you have one or more of these additional problems, you should give particular attention to reducing your risk.
* If you are a woman under 45 years or a man under 35 years of age, your RISKO score represents an upper limit on your real risk of developing heart disease. In this case your real risk is probably lower than indicated by your score.
* If you are a woman whose use of estrogen has contributed to a high RISKO score, you may want to consult your physician. Do not automatically discontinue your prescription.
* Using your weight category to estimate your systolic blood pressure or your blood cholesterol level makes your RISKO score less accurate.
  * Your score will tend to overestimate your risk if your actual values on these two important factors are average for someone of your height and weight.
  * Your score will underestimate your risk if your actual blood pressure or cholesterol level is above average for someone of your height or weight.

UNDERSTANDING HEART DISEASE

In the United States it is estimated that close to 550,000 people die each year from coronary heart disease. Coronary artery disease is the most common type of heart disease and the leading cause of death in the United States and many other countries.

Coronary heart disease is the result of coronary atherosclerosis. Coronary atherosclerosis is the name of the process by which an accumulation of fatty deposits leads to a thickening and narrowing of the inner walls of the arteries that carry oxygenated blood and nutrients to the heart muscle. The effect is similar to that of a water pipe clogged by deposits.

The resulting restriction of the blood supply to the heart muscle can cause injury to the muscle as well as angina (chest pain). If the restriction of the blood supply is severe or if it continues over a period of time, the heart muscle cells fed by the restricted artery suffer irreversible injury and die. This is known as a myocardial infarction or heart attack.

Scientists have identified a number of factors which are linked with an increased likelihood or risk of developing coronary heart disease. Some of these risk factors, like aging, being male, or having a family history of heart disease, are unavoidable. However, many other significant risk factors, including all of the factors used to determine your RISKO score, can be changed to reduce the likelihood of developing heart disease.

APPRAISING YOUR RISK

- The RISKO heart hazard appraisal is an indicator of risk for adults who do not currently show evidence of heart disease. However, if you already have heart disease, it is very important that you work with your doctor in reducing your risk.
- The original concept of RISKO was developed by the Michigan Heart Association.
- It has been further developed by the American Heart Association with the assistance of Drs. John and Sonja McKinlay in Boston. It is based on the Framingham, Stanford, and Chicago heart disease studies. The format of RISKO was tested and refined by Dr. Robert M. Chamberlain and Dr. Armin Weinberg of the National Heart Center at the Baylor College of Medicine in Houston.

- RISKO scores are based upon four of the most important modifiable factors which contribute to the development of heart disease. These factors include your weight, blood pressure, blood cholesterol level, and use of tobacco. If you are a woman, your score will also take into account your use of estrogen.
- The RISKO score you obtain measures your risk of developing heart disease in the next several years, provided that you currently show no evidence of such disease.
- The RISKO heart hazard appraisal is not a substitute for a thorough physical examination and assessment by your physician. Rather, it will help you learn more about your risk of developing heart disease and will indicate ways in which you can reduce this risk.

AMERICAN CANCER SOCIETY GENERAL HEALTH STATUS INVENTORY

In development for potential release in 1989 by the American Cancer Society is an early detection educational effort focusing on the family. It will address cancer tests, risk factors, and symptoms in an easily comprehended format. The assessment inventory will assist in conveying the message to the public that the early detection of cancer requires a partnership between the individual and the health practitioner. Below is a draft example of the type of statements which are being considered for use in the assessment form. Note how there is an interconnection of skin cancer issues across the three categories of cancer tests, risk factors, and symptoms.

Cancer Tests: _____ Full body skin exam at all ages, especially checking moles (ask your doctor how to do a skin self exam at home)

Risk Factors: _____ Periodic overexposure to sunlight or tanning lamps

Symptoms: _____ Sore that does not heal
Change in mole

For additional information about this inventory, contact your ACS Division office, or write to the American Cancer Society, Department of Public Education, Tower Place, 3340 Peachtree Road, N.E., Atlanta, GA 30026.

Printed with the permission of the American Cancer Society

Operation Lifestyle

Your Lifestyle Profile

Mission Vraie-Vie
Votre Profil-Vie

Health and Welfare Canada

Santé et Bien-être social Canada

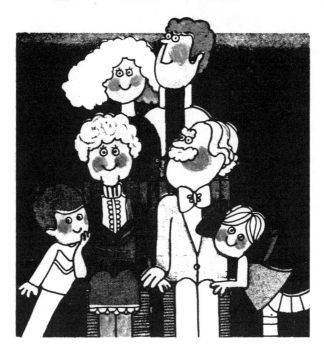

Reprinted with permission of Health and Welfare Canada

Operation Lifestyle

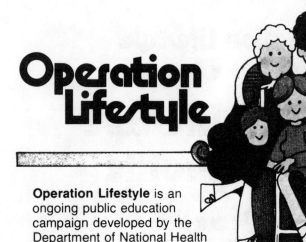

Operation Lifestyle is an ongoing public education campaign developed by the Department of National Health and Welfare to encourage Canadians to preserve their health through improved lifestyle habits. Start your new **Lifestyle** strategy today.

Lifestyle is the unique pattern of your daily life.

Lifestyle is neither sickness nor health. It is the food you eat, the weight problem, the malnutrition, the balanced diet.

Lifestyle is the vehicle you drive, the seatbelts you don't wear, the speed limits you choose to disobey.

Lifestyle is the drugs you take, the cigarettes you smoke, the alcohol you drink. It is addiction and moderation… it's abuse of over-the-counter drugs, use of illegal drugs and it's intelligent use of medication.

Lifestyle is becoming fit and staying that way through regular physical activity, or it's running to seed. It's participating in sports or being an observer, pursuing a hobby or watching television.

Lifestyle is how you handle stress, tension, and loneliness… it's knowing how to relax.

Lifestyle is taking precautions or needless risks with your health, on the job, at home, at school or while participating in sports.

Your Lifestyle Profile

— Indicate by circling or checking only the coloured signs that apply to you.
— The plus (+) and minus (−) signs next to some numbers indicate more than (+) and less than (−).

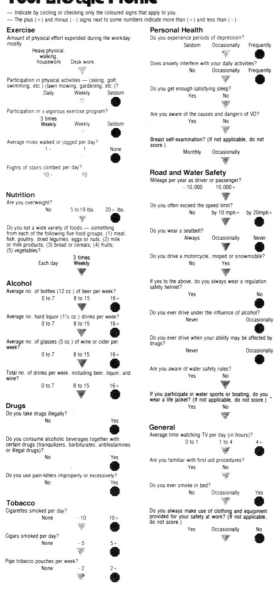

Exercise

Amount of physical effort expended during the workday: mostly

Heavy physical, walking, housework	Desk work
	▽

Participation in physical activities — (skiing, golf, swimming, etc.) (lawn mowing, gardening, etc.)?

Daily	Weekly	Seldom
	▽	●

Participation in a vigorous exercise program?

3 times Weekly	Weekly	Seldom
	▽	●

Average miles walked or jogged per day?

1 −	1	None
	▽	●

Flights of stairs climbed per day?

10 −	10
	●

Nutrition

Are you overweight?

No	5 to 19 lbs.	20+ lbs.
	▽	●

Do you eat a wide variety of foods — something from each of the following five food groups: (1) meat, fish, poultry, dried legumes, eggs or nuts; (2) milk or milk products; (3) bread or cereals; (4) fruits; (5) vegetables?

Each day	3 times Weekly
	▽

Alcohol

Average no. of bottles (12 oz.) of beer per week?

0 to 7	8 to 15	16+
	▽	●

Average no. hard liquor (1½ oz.) drinks per week?

0 to 7	8 to 15	16+
	▽	●

Average no. of glasses (5 oz.) of wine or cider per week?

0 to 7	8 to 15	16+
	▽	●

Total no. of drinks per week, including beer, liquor, and wine?

0 to 7	8 to 15	16+
	▽	●

Drugs

Do you take drugs illegally?

No	Yes
	●

Do you consume alcoholic beverages together with certain drugs (tranquilizers, barbiturates, antihistamines or illegal drugs)?

No	Yes
	●

Do you use pain-killers improperly or excessively?

No	Yes
	●

Tobacco

Cigarettes smoked per day?

None	−10	10+
	▽	●

Cigars smoked per day?

None	−5	5+
	▽	●

Pipe tobacco pouches per week?

None	−2	2+
	▽	●

Personal Health

Do you experience periods of depression?

Seldom	Occasionally	Frequently
	▽	●

Does anxiety interfere with your daily activities?

No	Occasionally	Frequently
		●

Do you get enough satisfying sleep?

Yes	No
	▽

Are you aware of the causes and dangers of VD?

Yes	No
	▽

Breast self-examination? (If not applicable, do not score.)

Monthly	Occasionally
	▽

Road and Water Safety

Mileage per year as driver or passenger?

−10,000	10,000+
	▽

Do you often exceed the speed limit?

No	by 10 mph+	by 20mph+
	▽	●

Do you wear a seatbelt?

Always	Occasionally	Never
	▽	●

Do you drive a motorcycle, moped or snowmobile?

No	Yes
	▽

If yes to the above, do you always wear a regulation safety helmet?

Yes	No
	●

Do you ever drive under the influence of alcohol?

Never	Occasionally
	●

Do you ever drive when your ability may be affected by drugs?

Never	Occasionally
	●

Are you aware of water safety rules?

Yes	No
	▽

If you participate in water sports or boating, do you wear a life jacket? (If not applicable, do not score.)

Yes	No
	▽

General

Average time watching TV per day (in hours)?

0 to 1	1 to 4	4+
	▽	●

Are you familiar with first-aid procedures?

Yes	No
	▽

Do you ever smoke in bed?

No	Occasionally	Yes
	▽	●

Do you always make use of clothing and equipment provided for your safety at work? (If not applicable, do not score.)

Yes	Occasionally	No
	▽	●

Sub totals				Sub totals			

Scoring Section

Count total number of ● 1 point for each   ▽ 3 points for each   ● 5 points for each   ● Your total score

Turn the page to see how you scored

How to calculate
your score

Excellent 34 - 45

Congratulations! "Excellent" indicates that
you have a commendable lifestyle based on
sensible habits and a lively awareness of
personal health. Keep up the good work and
maintain this rating.

Good 46 - 55

You have a sound grasp of basic health
principles. Only one to ten points separate
you from the elite. With a minimum of change
you can develop an excellent lifestyle
pattern. Make the effort to move up to
"Excellent" and stay there.

Risky 56 - 65

You are taking unnecessary risks with your
health. Several of your lifestyle habits are
based on unwise personal choices which
should be changed if potential health
problems are to be avoided. Look at your test
again. Start your improvements with the
places you lost points. A few common-sense
decisions can mean a "Good" rating, but the
challenge is to move your lifestyle up to
"Excellent".

Hazardous 66 and over

A "Hazardous" rating indicates a high risk
lifestyle. Either you have little personal
awareness of good health habits, or you are
choosing to ignore them. This is a danger
zone — but even hazardous lifestyles can be
modified and potential health problems
overcome. All it takes is a little conscientious
effort to improve basic living patterns. Go
over your test carefully and start making
those improvements right now.

Whether good or bad your **lifestyle** is what you make it. It *will change according to your attitude and ability to change*. To help you determine the quality of your own **lifestyle**, the Department of National Health and Welfare has developed the **Lifestyle Profile**.

The **Lifestyle Profile** will indicate where **lifestyle** changes should be made; but only if you answer the questions as objectively as possible.

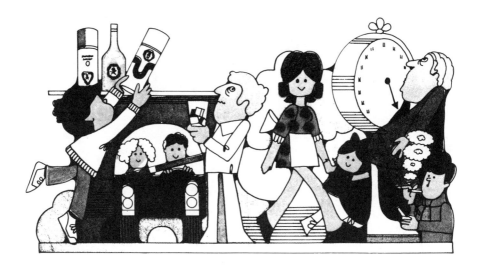

SELF-SCORING STRESS TEST

BEHAVIOUR

(Circle a number for each statement and add up your own score)	ALMOST ALWAYS	A FEW TIMES A WEEK	RARELY
1. I feel tense, anxious, or have nervous indigestion.	2	1	0
2. I seem to be low in energy.	2	1	0
3. I eat/drink/smoke in response to tension.	2	1	0
4. I have tension or migraine headaches, or pain in the neck or shoulders.	2	1	0
5. I seem to have trouble getting to sleep naturally or have difficulty getting back to sleep if awakened.	2	1	0
6. I find it difficult to concentrate on what I'm doing because of worrying about other things.	2	1	0
7. I take pills, medicine, alcohol, marijuana or other drugs to relax.	2	1	0
8. I have difficulty finding enough time to relax.	2	1	0
9. If I finally find the time, it is hard for me to relax.	2	1	0
10. I feel pressured during my workday.	2	1	0
11. I find it difficult to laugh.	2	1	0

Maximum total score = 22

My total score = _____
　　　　　　　　　　now　　　3 months from now　　　6 months from now

Today's Date _____

_____

From: *Your Way to Wellness Workbook*, Evalu-Life, Health and Welfare Canada. Reprinted with permission.

Appendix B
"Healthier People" Health Risk Appraisal

THE
CARTER CENTER
OF EMORY UNIVERSITY

Healthier People
Health Risk Appraisal

Nº 15428

Detach this coupon and put it in a safe place.
You will need it to claim your appraisal results.

- -

Healthier People
Health Risk Appraisal
The Carter Center of Emory University

Nº 15428

Health Risk Appraisal is an educational tool. It shows you choices you can make to keep good health and avoid the most common causes of death for a person your age and sex. This Health Risk Appraisal is not a substitute for a check-up or physical exam that you get from a doctor or nurse. It only gives you some ideas for lowering your risk of getting sick or injured in the future. It is NOT designed for people who already have HEART DISEASE, CANCER, KIDNEY DISEASE, OR OTHER SERIOUS CONDITIONS. If you have any of these problems and you want a Health Risk Appraisal anyway, ask your doctor or nurse to read the report with you.
DIRECTIONS: To keep your answers confidential DO NOT write your name or any identification on this form. Please keep the coupon with your participant number on it. You will need it to claim your computer report. To get the most accurate results answer as many questions as you can and as best you can. If you do not know the answer leave it blank. Questions with a ★ (star symbol) are important to your health, but are not used by the computer to calculate your risks. However, your answers may be helpful in planning your health and fitness program. **Note:** This Health Risk Appraisal form is still being tested and improved. It may have mistakes or errors in it. If anything in your questionnaire or report doesn't seem right to you, ask a health person to help.

Please put your answers in the empty boxes. (Examples: ⊠ or 125)

1. SEX	1 ☐ Male 2 ☐ Female
2. AGE	☐ Years
3. HEIGHT (Without shoes) (No fractions)	☐ Feet ☐ Inches
4. WEIGHT (Without shoes) (No fractions)	☐ Pounds
5. Body frame size	1 ☐ Small 2 ☐ Medium 3 ☐ Large
6. Have you ever been told that you have diabetes (or sugar diabetes)?	1 ☐ Yes 2 ☐ No
7. Are you now taking medicine for high blood pressure?	1 ☐ Yes 2 ☐ No
8. What is your blood pressure now?	☐ / ☐ Systolic (High number) / Diastolic (Low number)
9. If you *do not* know the numbers, check the box that describes your blood pressure.	1 ☐ High 2 ☐ Normal or Low 3 ☐ Don't Know
10. What is your TOTAL cholesterol level (based on a blood test)?	☐ mg/dl
11. What is your HDL cholesterol (based on a blood test)?	☐ mg/dl
12. How many cigars do you usually smoke per day?	☐ cigars per day
13. How many pipes of tobacco do you usually smoke per day?	☐ pipes per day
14. How many times per day do you usually use smokeless tobacco? (Chewing tobacco, snuff, pouches, etc.)	☐ times per day

Reprinted with the permission of Health Risk Appraisal Program, The Carter Center, Emory University

APPENDICES   163

Health Risk Appraisal is an educational tool. It shows you choices you can make to keep good health and avoid the most common causes of death for a person your age and sex. This Health Risk Appraisal is not a substitute for a check-up or physical exam that you get from a doctor or nurse. It only gives you some ideas for lowering your risk of getting sick or injured in the future. It is NOT designed for people who already have HEART DISEASE, CANCER, KIDNEY DISEASE, OR OTHER SERIOUS CONDITIONS. If you have any of these problems and you want a Health Risk Appraisal anyway, ask your doctor or nurse to read the report with you.

Your report may be picked up at _____ on _____.   (D)

---

15. CIGARETTE SMOKING
How would you describe your cigarette smoking habits?

1 ☐ Never smoked ☛ Go to 18
2 ☐ Used to smoke ☛ Go to 17
3 ☐ Still smoke ☛ Go to 16

16. STILL SMOKE
How many cigarettes a day do you smoke?

[ ] cigarettes per day ☛ Go to 18

17. USED TO SMOKE
a. How many years has it been since you smoked cigarettes fairly regularly?

[ ] years

b. What was the average number of cigarettes per day that you smoked in the 2 years before you quit?

[ ] cigarettes per day

---

18. In the next 12 months how many thousands of miles will you probably travel by each of the following? (NOTE: U.S. average = 10,000 miles)
   a. Car, truck, or van:
   b. Motorcycle:

[ ],000 miles
[ ],000 miles

---

19. On a typical day how do you USUALLY travel?

(Check one only)

1 ☐ Walk
2 ☐ Bicycle
3 ☐ Motorcycle
4 ☐ Sub-compact or compact car
5 ☐ Mid-size or full-size car
6 ☐ Truck or van
7 ☐ Bus, subway, or train
8 ☐ Mostly stay home

---

20. What percent of the time do you usually buckle your safety belt when driving or riding?

[ ] %

---

21. On the average, how close to the speed limit do you usually drive?

1 ☐ Within 5 mph of limit
2 ☐ 6-10 mph over limit
3 ☐ 11-15 mph over limit
4 ☐ More than 15 mph over limit

---

22. How many times in the last month did you drive or ride when the driver had perhaps too much alcohol to drink?

[ ] times last month

---

23. How many drinks of alcoholic beverages do you have in a typical week?

☛ (MEN GO TO QUESTION 33)

(Write the number of each type of drink)
[ ] Bottles or cans of beer
[ ] Glasses of wine
[ ] Wine coolers
[ ] Mixed drinks or shots of liquor

WOMEN
24. At what age did you have your first menstrual period?

[ ] years old

---

25. How old were you when your first child was born?

[ ] years old
(If no children write 0)

26. How long has it been since your last breast x-ray (mammogram)?	1 ☐ Less than 1 year ago 2 ☐ 1 year ago 3 ☐ 2 years ago 4 ☐ 3 or more years ago 5 ☐ Never
27. How many women in your natural family (mother and sisters only) have had breast cancer?	☐ women
28. Have you had a hysterectomy operation?	1 ☐ Yes 2 ☐ No 3 ☐ Not sure
29. How long has it been since you had a pap smear for cancer?	1 ☐ Less than 1 year ago 2 ☐ 1 year ago 3 ☐ 2 years ago 4 ☐ 3 or more years ago 5 ☐ Never
★ 30. How often do you examine your breasts for lumps.	1 ☐ Monthly 2 ☐ Once every few months 3 ☐ Rarely or never
★ 31. About how long has it been since you had your breasts examined by a physician or nurse?	1 ☐ Less than 1 year ago 2 ☐ 1 year ago 3 ☐ 2 years ago 4 ☐ 3 or more years ago 5 ☐ Never
★ 32. About how long has it been since you had a rectal exam? ☞ *(WOMEN GO TO QUESTION 34)*	1 ☐ Less than 1 year ago 2 ☐ 1 year ago 3 ☐ 2 years ago 4 ☐ 3 or more years ago 5 ☐ Never
MEN ★ 33. About how long has it been since you had a rectal or prostate exam?	1 ☐ Less than 1 year ago 2 ☐ 1 year ago 3 ☐ 2 years ago 4 ☐ 3 or more years ago 5 ☐ Never
★ 34. How many times in the last year did you witness or become involved in a violent fight or attack where there was a good chance of a serious injury to someone?	1 ☐ 4 or more times 2 ☐ 2 or 3 times 3 ☐ 1 time or never 4 ☐ Not sure
★ 35. Considering your age, how would you describe your overall physical health?	1 ☐ Excellent 2 ☐ Good 3 ☐ Fair 4 ☐ Poor
★ 36. In an average week, how many times do you engage in physical activity (exercise or work which lasts at least 20 minutes without stopping and which is hard enough to make you breathe heavier and your heart beat faster)?	1 ☐ Less than 1 time per week 2 ☐ 1 or 2 times per week 3 ☐ At least 3 times per week
★ 37. If you ride a motorcycle or all-terrain vehicle (ATV) what percent of the time do you wear a helmet?	1 ☐ 75% to 100% 2 ☐ 25% to 74% 3 ☐ Less than 25% 4 ☐ Does not apply to me

★ 38. Do you eat some food every day that is high in fiber, such as whole grain bread, cereal, fresh fruits or vegetables?	1 ☐ Yes	2 ☐ No

★ 39. Do you eat foods every day that are high in cholesterol or fat, such as fatty meat, cheese, fried foods, or eggs?	1 ☐ Yes	2 ☐ No

★ 40. In general, how satisfied are you with your life?

1 ☐ Mostly satisfied
2 ☐ Partly satisfied
3 ☐ Not satisfied

★ 41. Have you suffered a personal loss or misfortune in the past year that had a serious impact on your life? (For example, a job loss, disability, separation, jail term, or the death of someone close to you.)

1 ☐ Yes, 1 serious loss or misfortune
2 ☐ Yes, 2 or more
3 ☐ No

★ 42a. Race

1 ☐ Aleutian, Alaska native, Eskimo or American Indian
2 ☐ Asian
3 ☐ Black
4 ☐ Pacific Islander
5 ☐ White
6 ☐ Other
7 ☐ Don't know

★ 42b. Are you of Hispanic origin such as Mexican-American, Puerto Rican, or Cuban?

1 ☐ Yes   2 ☐ No

★ 43. What is the highest grade you completed in school?

1 ☐ Grade school or less
2 ☐ Some high school
3 ☐ High school graduate
4 ☐ Some college
5 ☐ College graduate
6 ☐ Post graduate or professional degree

★ 44. What is your job or occupation?

(Check only one)

1 ☐ Health professional
2 ☐ Manager, educator, professional
3 ☐ Technical, sales or administrative support
4 ☐ Operator, fabricator, laborer
5 ☐ Student
6 ☐ Retired
7 ☐ Homemaker
8 ☐ Service
9 ☐ Skilled crafts
10 ☐ Unemployed
11 ☐ Other

★ 45. In what industry do you work (or did you) last work?

(Check only one)

1 ☐ Electric, gas, sanitation
2 ☐ Transportation, communication
3 ☐ Agriculture, forestry, fishing
4 ☐ Wholesale or retail trade
5 ☐ Financial and service industries
6 ☐ Mining
7 ☐ Government
8 ☐ Manufacturing
9 ☐ Construction
10 ☐ Other

Ⓓ

Sample HRA Printout

<pre>
                          Healthier People
              The Carter Center of Emory University
578368   Atlanta, Georgia   Tue Nov 10 1987
Male Age 47   Version C-87
              ....
              | YOUR   NOW   TARGET |
              | RISK AGE: 46.92 years   41.08 years |
              ....
</pre>

Many serious injuries and health problems can be prevented. Your Health Risk Appraisal lists factors you can change to lower your risk. For causes of death that are not directly computable, the report uses the average risk for persons of your age and sex. More technical detail about the report is on page 2.

MOST COMMON CAUSES OF DEATH	NUMBER OF DEATHS IN NEXT 10 YEARS FOR 1000 MEN AGE 47			RISK FACTORS YOU CAN CHANGE
	YOUR RISK	RISK TARGET	AVERAGE RISK	
Heart Attack	30	12	24	Avoid Tobacco Use, Blood Pressure, Cholesterol Level, HDL Level, Weight
Lung Cancer	10	4	9	Avoid Tobacco Use
Stroke	4	2	3	Avoid Tobacco Use, Blood Pressure
Motor Vehicle Crash	4	1	2	Reduce Speeding, Wear Seat Belts
Suicide	2*	2*	2	Get Help from a Health Professional if Needed
Emphysema/Bronchitis	2	<1	1	Avoid Tobacco Use
Other Injuries	2*	2*	2	Avoid Heavy Alcohol Use and Observe Safety Rules
Cirrhosis of Liver	2	2	4	Continue to Avoid Heavy Drinking
Homicide	2*	2*	2	Avoid Drug/Alcohol Use and Handguns
Colon Cancer	2*	2*	2	A High-Fiber and Low-Fat Diet Might Reduce Risk
Esophagus Cancer	2	<1	1	Avoid Tobacco Use
All Other	31	29	32	
	....	....	....	* = Average Value Used
TOTAL:	90	58	83	Deaths in Next 10 Years Per 1,000 MEN, Age 47

| For Height 5'11" and Medium Frame, 182 pounds is about 17% Overweight. Desirable Weight Range: 147-162 |

GOOD HABITS	TO IMPROVE YOUR RISK PROFILE:	RISK YEARS GAINED
+ Low alcohol risk	- Quit smoking	3.48
+ You don't use smokeless tobacco	- Lower your cholesterol	1.12
	- Improve HDL level	0.44
	- Reduce driving speed to legal limit	0.28
	- Always wear your seat belts	0.25
	- Lower your blood pressure	0.16
	- Bring your weight to desirable range	0.10

Total Risk Years you could gain = 5.84

APPENDICES 167

578368
Male Age 47

```
........................................        ........................................
|   ROUTINE PREVENTIVE SERVICES FOR MEN YOUR AGE  |      |   GENERAL RECOMMENDATIONS FOR EVERYONE   |
|                                                 |      |                                          |
| Blood Pressure and Cholesterol test            |      | * Exercise briskly for 15 - 30 minutes   |
| Prostate/Rectal exam (or Sigmoidoscopy)        |      |   at least three times a week             |
| Eye exam for glaucoma                           |      | * Use good eating habits by choosing a    |
| Dental exam                                     |      |   variety of foods that are low in fat    |
| Tetanus-Diphtheria booster shot (every 10 years)|      |   and cholesterol and high in fiber       |
|                                                 |      | * Learn to recognize and handle stress -  |
|                                                 |      |   get help if you need it                 |
........................................        ........................................
```

ADDITIONAL REPORT FROM: The Carter Center of Emory University

PLEASE NOTE: This computer program is VERSION 0.3 of the HRA. It is still being tested.

ADDITIONAL MESSAGE FROM: The Carter Center of Emory University

Many Americans are concerned about the risk of getting AIDS. AIDS is caused by a virus that is spread by sexual
contact and by sharing needles during drug use. AIDS may also be passed from a mother to an unborn child during
pregnancy or at birth. A small number of cases of AIDS were caused by blood transfusions received between 1977
and 1985. The blood supply is now quite safe because of screening programs. AIDS is not spread by day to day
contact such as being near, touching, or eating with a person with AIDS. There is no vaccine or cure, but AIDS
can be prevented. For further information call the AIDS Hotline: 1-800-342-AIDS (2437).

ABOUT THIS REPORT

This Health Risk Appraisal is different from a check-up or a health exam that you would get from a doctor or a
nurse. It cannot tell if you are sick or have a medical problem. It only gives you some ideas for lowering your
risks of getting sick or injured in the future.

Average rates are based on United States death certificate data, and reflect current health patterns, medical
practices and environmental conditions. Appraised rates (YOUR RISK) are computed for persons with your current
health and safety practices. Achievable rates (RISK TARGET) are computed for persons who can reduce risk factors
to a lower level. All of the risks are computed from data of the Carter Center Health Risk Appraisal Project,
with technical support of the Centers for Disease Control and 20 other major health agencies.

CAUTION: This computer program is still being tested. It may have mistakes or errors in it. If anything in your
printout doesn't seem right to you, ask your interpreter to check your printout. Since it is a developmental
program, it should be interpreted by a qualified health professional.

For additional information please write: Health Risk Appraisal Program
                                          The Carter Center of Emory University
                                          1989 N. Williamsburg Drive, Suite E
                                          Atlanta, Georgia 30033

Reprinted with the permission of Health Risk Appraisal Program, The Carter Center, Emory University

Appendix C
La Crosse Wellness Project

LA CROSSE WELLNESS INVENTORY (LWI)

Below is a sampling of two statements from each of the NINE sections in the LWI. There is a total of 183 statements in the LWI. Scoring by computer and a printout are available for a minimum charge. Software may be purchased or leased.

SAMPLE OF INVENTORY STATEMENTS FROM NINE WELLNESS CATEGORIES

1. **REST AND RELAXATION**

   I engage in nervous habits (e.g., biting or picking my fingernails).
   I am able to relax my mind and body without the use of drugs.

2. **EMOTIONAL AND MENTAL HEALTH**

   I can accept constructive criticism without reacting defensively.
   I feel good about myself even when I make mistakes.

3. **PERSONAL HABITS**

   I floss my teeth daily.
   I seek medical attention when experiencing early signs and symptoms of illness.

4. **FITNESS**

   I have my blood pressure checked at least once a year.
   I consider myself overweight.

5. **NUTRITION**

   I drink more than 4 cups of beverages containing caffeine per day (coffee, tea, cocoa).
   I read ingredient labels on packaged foods.

6. **DRUGS**

   I am aware of the major side effects that could occur with the prescribed medications that I take.
   I need alcohol to be sociable.

7. **SAFETY**

   I wear a safety belt and/or shoulder harness when in a vehicle.
   There are smoke detectors in my place of residence.

8. **ENVIRONMENTAL SENSITIVITY**

   My (our) household uses non-polluting detergents.
   I am aware that recycling materials is important.

9. **SEXUALITY**

   I am satisfied with the sexual part of my life.
   My sexual activity is consistant with my sexual beliefs and values.

Wellness Development Process (WDP): Intervention and Reinforcement

The following pages provide a brief sample of the Process Workbook Contents. These pages should help clarify the "process" an individual experiences developing intervention strategies and reinforcements.

PREFACE

Welcome to the Wellness Development Process of the La Crosse Wellness Project (LWP). Earlier you completed the La Crosse Wellness Inventory, which was the Assessment stage. Now you have the opportunity to go through the Intervention and Reinforcement stages of wellness. In these stages, you will examine your current level of wellness and establish a process for wellness enhancement in your life.

There are several points that we would like to make before you continue. Please notice that we have made every effort in this project to stay away from establishing the kind of scoring system which forces you to compare yourself with others. While we believe that "comparing ourselves to others" is one way of valuing our lives, we also believe that people should learn how to value themselves. This means comparing yourself with yourself, rather than constantly comparing yourself to the expectations of society. As a result, we have designed an inventory which encourages you to assess yourself and then to make decisions about your assessment. This provides you with the basis to make some plans for your lifestyle choices.

Your potential for an improved lifestyle corresponds to your investment in reading the Wellness Development Process booklet and your investment in understanding the process. We recognize that this booklet is lengthy. Its structure provides you with educational and conceptual information on the left side and a worksheet to the right. We highly recommend that you take the time to read the information on the left before completing the worksheet to the right.

The Wellness Development Process, contained in this booklet, consists of four sections:
  1) Establishing a Wellness Area for Enhancement
  2) Identifying Wellness Outcomes
  3) Establishing Wellness Activities
  4) Working Toward Personal Enhancement

Their order and content are designed to foster specific understanding of how to make changes in your life. The purpose of the LWP is to help you learn how to:
  1) assess your life;
  2) select areas for enhancement;
  3) establish activities for enhancement;
  4) establish rewards for enhancement;

Wellness involves a life-long learning process in which health-related decisions are made to maximize your health promotion potential. Health promotion is a way of life and the responsibility belongs to each of us.

You will get out of this development process what you choose to put into it.

> Margaret F. Dosch
> Gary D. Gilmore
> Thomas L. Hood
>
> Steering Committee Members
> for the La Crosse Wellness Project
> 203 Mitchell Hall
> University of Wisconsin–La Crosse
> La Crosse, WI 54601

**Enhancement
Moving Toward Total Wellness**

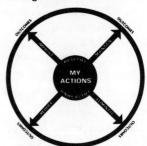

Enhancement means reducing or eliminating unhealthy actions in your life, and/or maintaining or improving healthy actions in your life. As you prepare to take your action steps, examine the figure on this page so that you can visualize the enhancement process.

Appendix D
Available Health Risk Appraisals and Wellness Inventories

Available Health Risk Appraisals and Wellness Inventories.

Title	Scoring Process	Description	Contact
Compuhealth	Mainframe Computer	Developed for corporations; Calculates costs and savings related to employee health	Overman Associates P. O. Box 171 Bonne Terre, MO 63628 Tel.: (314) 562-7020
General Well-Being Questionnaire	Mainframe Computer	Emphasizes current levels of fitness rather than future disease	Healthline St. Louis Univ. Medical Center 1325 South Grand Boulevard St. Louis, MO 63104 Tel.: (314) 771-7601
Health Age	Microcomputer	Information on seven health habits; computes a health age in contrast to chronological age	Wellsource 15431 S.E. 82nd Drive Suite E PO Box 569 Clackamas, OR 97015 Tel.: (503) 656-7446
Health and Lifestyle Questionnaire	Mainframe Computer	Emphasizes current quality of life over long-term risks	Health Enhancement Systems 9 Mercer Street Princeton, NJ 08540 Tel.: (609) 924-7799

Title	Scoring Process	Description	Contact
Health Awareness Games	Microcomputer	Statistics about lifestyle and health as they relate to life expectancy	HRM Software 175 Tompkins Avenue Pleasantville, NY 10570 Tel.: (914) 769-6900
Health Hazard Appraisal	Mainframe Computer	Statistically updated version of the original HRA developed at Methodist Hospital	Prospective Medicine Center Suite 219 3901 North Meridian Indianapolis, IN 46208 Tel.: (317) 923-3600
Health Hazard Appraisal Questionnaire	Mainframe Computer	Personal and family medical history; also includes sections on alcohol, smoking and driving; special section for women	University of California Dept. of Epidemiology & International Health 1699 HSW San Francisco, CA 94143 Tel.: (415) 476-1158
Health Maintenance Volume II	Microcomputer	Developed for high school students; first program is an interactive HRA, second concerns ideal weight	MECC Distribution Center Minnesota Educational Computing Consortium (MECC) 3490 Lexington Avenue North St. Paul, MN 55112 Tel.: (612) 481-3527
Health Risk Appraisal	Mainframe Computer	Covers health habits and medical status	University of Michigan Fitness Research Center 401 Washtenaw Avenue Ann Arbor, MI 48109 Tel.: (313) 763-2462
Health Risk Appraisal	Microcomputer	Interactive HRA on lifestyle and physiological indicators	University of Minnesota Media Distribution Box 734, Mayo Building 420 Delaware Street, S.E. Minneapolis, MN 55455 Tel.: (612) 624-7906

Name	Type	Description	Contact
Health Risk Appraisal Questionnaire	Mainframe Computer	Covers personal and family medical history, health habits, and women's health	St. Louis County Health Department 504 East Second Street Duluth, MN 55805 Tel.: (218) 727-8661
Health Risk Assessment Questionnaire	Mainframe Computer	Emphasizes premature mortality risk factors including medical history, physical examination, family history, and personal health habits	Wisconsin Center for Health Risk Research University of Wisconsin Center for Health Sciences 600 Highland Avenue, Room J5/224 Madison, WI 53792 Tel.: (608) 263-9530
Health Risk Profile	Mainframe Computer	Emphasizes medical and family history; health habits and lifestyles, particularly stress factors, are also covered	Control Data Corporation Benefit Services Division 8800 Queen Avenue South PO Box 1305 Minneapolis, MN 55440 Tel.: (612) 921-6542 (800) 853-7777
Health Risk Profile for Life and Health Enhancement	Mainframe Computer	AN HRA originally developed for low income populations in an urban setting, this process is now used in clinic and outreach efforts	Division of Health Education Milwaukee City Health Department 841 North Broadway Milwaukee, WI 53202 Tel.: (414) 278-3635
Health Risk Questionnaire	Mainframe Computer	Emphasizes lifestyle, medical history, and some physical and laboratory measurements	Health Enhancement Systems 9 Mercer Street Princeton, NJ 08540 Tel.: (609) 924-7799
Health Status Profile	Mainframe Computer	Collects information on current symptoms, medications used, and medical history and probes nutrition, stress, and exercise habits	Health Enhancement Systems 9 Mercer Street Princeton, NJ 08540 Tel.: (609) 924-7799

Title	Scoring Process	Description	Contact
Healthcheck	Microcomputer	Developed for field workers; covers nutrition, stress, and exercise, as well as medical and family history and women's health	American Wellness System, Inc. 6000 Lake Forrest Drive N.W. Suite 255 Atlanta, GA 30328 Tel.: (404) 256-9366 (800) 832-9355
Healthier People Health Risk Appraisal	Mainframe and Microcomputer	Emphasizes lowering of health risks of future sickness or illness	Health Risk Appraisal Project[1] The Carter Center Emory University 1989 North Williamsburg Drive Suite E Decatur, GA 30033 Tel.: (404) 321-4104
Healthline	Mainframe Computer	Data on medical history and lifestyle, women's health, stress, and psychological and social factors, exercise and nutrition	Health Logics PO Box 3430 San Leandro, CA 94578 Tel.: (415) 573-7222 (415) 341-1895
Healthplan	Mainframe Computer	Data on personal and family medical history; behavior habits, socioeconomic status, and women's health	General Health 3299 K Street, NW Washington, DC 20007 Tel.: (202) 965-4881 (800) 424-2775
Healthstyle	Microcomputer	Emphasizes personal health habits that influence one's health	Wellsource 15431 Southeast 82nd Drive Suite E Clackamas, OR 97015 Tel.: (503) 656-7446
Healthstyle: A Self-Test	Self-scored	Developed to explain how personal habits influence one's health; specific suggestions for reducing risks	ODPHP Health Information Center PO Box 1133 Washington, DC 20013 Tel.: (202) 429-9091 (800) 336-4797

Healthwrap	Mainframe Computer	Emphasizes questions of the CDC instrument plus questions on wellness	Lifestyle and Health Promotion PO box 2177 Boone, NC 28607 Tel.: (704) 264-2897 (704) 264-0674

[1] More specific contact information for the "Healthier People" HRA version.

State Contacts:

State	Contact	Phone	State	Contact	Phone
Alabama	James J. McVay	(205) 261-5095	Montana	Robert Moon	(406) 444-4740
Arizona	Mary Downs	(602) 255-1008	New Hampshire	Susan Sielke	(603) 271-4551
California	Frank Capell	(916) 322-4787	New Jersey	Steven Young	(609) 292-4728
Delaware	Frank Breukelman	(302) 736-4724	Ohio	Morris F. Stamm	(614) 466-4626
Florida	Marney Richards	(904) 488-2901	Oklahoma	Neil Hann	(405) 271-5601
Idaho	Joe Patterson	(208) 334-5929	South Carolina	Thomas F. Gillette	(803) 734-4790
Illinois	Darrell Patterson	(217) 785-2060	Tennessee	John Fortune	(615) 741-7366
Indiana	Mike Atkinson	(317) 633-0270	Texas	Juli Fellows	(512) 458-7405
Kentucky	Phyllis Skonicki	(502) 564-7112	Utah	Denise Basse	(801) 533-6120
Louisiana	Roland Batiste	(504) 568-5444	Virginia	Rod Hyner	(804) 786-3551
Maine	Michael T. Gay	(207) 289-3201	West Virginia	Robert H. Anderson	(304) 348-0644

States and territories not listed above may call one of the following:

Emory University — Martha E. Alexander — (404) 727-0262
Arkansas, Georgia, Kansas, Missouri, Mississippi, Nebraska, North Carolina, Puerto Rico, Virgin Islands

Johns Hopkins University — Maia Belosevic — (301) 955-8110
Connecticut, Iowa, Maryland, Massachusetts, Minnesota, New York, Pennsylvania, Rhode Island, Vermont, Washington, D.C., Wisconsin, Michigan

University of Northern Colorado — Mary Davis — (303) 351-2755
Alaska, Colorado, Guam, Hawaii, Nevada, New Mexico, North Dakota, Oregon, South Dakota, Washington, Wyoming

For information in Canada: Sylvie Bisson — (613) 990-7731

Inquiries from countries other than the U.S. and Canada:

David Moriarty — (404) 329-3452

Title	Scoring Process	Description	Contact
Heartchec	Microcomputer	Emphasizes eating habits, smoking, exercise, stress, and other lifestyle factors	Wellsource for Health and Fitness 15431 Southeast 82nd Drive Suite E PO Box 569 Clackamas, OR 97015 Tel.: (503) 656-7446
Hospitalization Risk Assessment Program	Microcomputer	Developed to assess hospitalization risks but relates only to those risks which an individual can modify	Tulane University Medical Center School of Public Health and Tropical Medicine Department of Health Systems Management 1501 Canal Street New Orleans, LA 70112 Tel.: (504) 588-5428
How Do You Rate As A Health Risk?	Self-scored	Emphasizes alcohol and other drugs, nutrition, weight control, exercise, stress and safety.	Channing L. Bete Co., Inc. 200 State Road South Deerfield, MA 01373 Tel.: (413) 665-7611
I'm A Health Nut	Microcomputer	Designed for adolescents; family and personal health data, lifestyles, feelings, and focus of control	St. Paul Division of Public Health Health Education Section 555 Cedar Street St. Paul, MN 55101 Tel.: (612) 292-7712
InnerView Health	Mainframe Computer	Utilizes machine readable questionnaires to gather input on individual lifestyles and health histories	National Computer Systems 11000 Prairie Lakes Drive Minneapolis, MN 55440 Tel.: (612) 830-8588
Is Your Body Older Than You Are?	Self-scored	Consists of same Blue Cross questionnaire used in *Determine Your Medical Age*	Blue Cross/Blue Shield of Oregon Corporate Communications 100 Southwest Market Street Portland, OR 97201 Tel.: (503) 255-5221

Name	Type	Description	Contact
La Crosse Wellness Project	Mainframe and Microcomputer	Emphasizes current levels of wellness with follow-up materials for planned change and reinforcement	La Crosse Wellness Project 203 Mitchell Hall University of Wisconsin-La Crosse La Crosse, WI 54601 Tel.: (608) 785-8162
Life	Mainframe Computer	Emphasizes personal and family medical histories, habits and lifestyle, attitudes to health, and physical measurements; diet exercise and other health-habits are explored	Wellsource 15431 Southeast 82nd Drive Suite E PO Box 569 Clackamas, OR 97015 Tel.: (503) 656-7446
Lifescan	Mainframe and Microcomputer	Emphasizes physical activity, drug usage, driving habits, cholesterol level, medical history, and women's health issues	National Wellness Institute University of Wisconsin-Stevens Point South Hall Stevens Point, WI 54481 Tel.: (715) 346-2172
Lifescore M	Microcomputer	Emphasizes habits and lifestyle, including environmental factors, utilization of health care, and family medical history	Center for Corporate Health Promotion 1850 Centennial Park Drive Suite 520 Reston, VA 22091 Tel.: (703) 391-1900
Lifescore Plus	Microcomputer	Based on biomedical measures (e.g., cholesterol levels, and blood pressure) lifestyle habits, and health history	Center for Corporate Health Promotion 1850 Centennial Park Drive Suite 520 Reston, VA 22091 Tel.: (703) 391-1900
Lifescore-C	Self-scored	Developed for employee health programs; covers lifestyle, environmental factors, family medical history, and utilization of health care	Center for Corporate Health Promotion 1850 Centennial Park Drive Suite 520 Reston, VA 22091 Tel.: (703) 391-1900

Title	Scoring Process	Description	Contact
Lifestyle Assessment Questionnaire (LAQ)	Mainframe Computer	Assesses the individual in six dimensions of wellness; personal growth section asks client to select topics to receive more information	National Wellness Institute University of Wisconsin-Stevens Point South Hall Stevens Point, WI 54481 Tel.: (715) 346-2172
Lifestyle Management System	Mainframe Computer	Developed to provide health and lifestyle information with positive feedback comparing an individual's health status to optimal status	Lifestyle Management Reports, Inc. 368 Congress Street Boston, MA 02210 Tel.: (800) 531-2348
Micro-HRA	Microcomputer	Developed at Leavenworth, Kansas, from which the CDC derived its HRA for micro-computers	Planetree Medical Systems 3519 South 1200 East #A Salt Lake City, UT 84106 Tel.: (801) 486-7640
Personal Health Appraisal	Microcomputers	Developed in "personal" and "professional" versions; personal version is interactive, while the professional version can be used in either interactive or batch-processing mode and can store and update profiles	MedMicro The Center for Medical Microcomputing PO Box 9615 Madison, WI 53715 Tel.: (608) 798-3002
Personal Health Inventory	Microcomputer	Emphasizes health habits, lifestyle, medical history, medical care, and women's health	American Corporate Health Programs Inc., (ACHP) 150 Strafford Avenue Suite 300 Wayne, PA 19087 Tel.: (215) 293-9367
Personal Health Profile	Mainframe	Collects demographic data and information on general well-being, stress, health status, and habits, including women's health	General Health 3299 K Street, NW Washington, DC 20007 Tel.: (202) 965-4881 (800) 424-2775

Personal Risk Profile	Mainframe Computer	Emphasizes personal and family medical history, the remainder on behavior, habits, socioeconomic status, and women's health	General Health, 3299 K Street, NW, Washington, DC 20007, Tel.: (202) 965-4881, (800) 424-2775
Pulse	Mainframe Computer	Emphasizes nutrition, exercise, stress, personal and family medical history, lifestyle, habits	International Health Awareness Center, 148 East Michigan Avenue, Kalamazoo, MI 49007, Tel.: (616) 343-0770, (800) 531-4076
RHRC Health Risk Appraisal	Mainframe and Microcomputers	Emphasizes the impact of workplace wellness programs	Regional Health Resource Center, Medical Information Laboratory, 1408 West University Avenue, Urbana, IL 61801, Tel.: (217) 367-0076
Sphere	Microcomputer	Developed in English and French, based on Canadian statistics; second English version based on U.S. statistics, covers medical and lifestyle characteristics	Care and Epidemiology, University of British Columbia, 5804 Fairview Crescent, Mather Building, Vancouver, BC V6T W5, Canada, Tel.: (604) 228-2258
Start Taking Charge	Self-scored	Emphasizes exercise, diet, safety, stress, and substance abuse	Aetna Life and Casualty, 151 Farmington Avenue, Hartford, CT 06156-MC17
Testwell	Microcomputer	Measures strength in social, occupational, spiritual, physical, intellectual, and emotional dimensions of wellness	National Wellness Institute, University of Wisconsin-Stevens Point, South Hall, Stevens Point, WI 54481, Tel.: (715) 346-2172

Title	Scoring Process	Description	Contact
Well Aware Health Risk Appraisal	Mainframe Computer	Developed under a 5-year Kellogg Foundation research grant, on health habits and lifestyle, health knowledge, stress, and women's health	Well Aware About Health PO Box 43338 Tucson, AZ 85733 Tel.: (602) 297-2819 Tel.: (602) 297-2960
Wellness Check	Mainframe and Microcomputer	Emphasizes health habits, family medical history, occupational exposure to hazardous substances, and women's health; adult and teen version available	Chief of Health Promotion Rhode Island Department of Health 75 Davis Street Providence, RI 02908 Tel.: (401) 277-6957
Wellness Index/Wellness Inventory	Self-scored	Assesses wellness in areas of personal energy expenditure emphasizing stress factors, personal relationships, and social attitudes	Wellness Associates Box 5433-H Mill Valley, CA 94942 Tel.: (415) 383-3806
Wellness Inventory —Interactive	Microcomputer	Emphasizes stress, personal relationships, and social attitudes	Wellness Associates Box 5433-H Mill Valley, CA 94942 Tel.: (415) 383-3806
Your Lifestyle Profile	Self-scored	Adapted from the Canadian quiz of the same name; one component of the Kansas PLUS employee health program	Kansas Department of Health and Environment Forbes Field Topeka, KS 66620 ATTN: Health Promotion PLUS Adm. Tel.: (913) 862-9360

Adapted from *Healthfinder: Health Risk Appraisals*, Office of Disease Prevention and Health Information, DHHS; 1987.

Appendix E
Community Risk Estimation

COMMUNITY ESTIMATION
by
Harriet H. Imrey, Ph.D.*

Community risk estimation is a natural outgrowth of individual health risk appraisal. It depends upon the same basic sciences of public health—epidemiology and biostatistics—and can be done with more or less attention to the basic rules of evidence and statistical rigor. Barring serious biases in the selection of risk factors and relative risks for the model, a community risk appraisal is likely to be more accurate than an individual appraisal because one can use the law of large numbers as a security blanket.

We are hearing more about community risk estimation in public health circles than we used to. Risk reduction programs in the public sector must demonstrate an effect upon public health in order to justify public support. Community risk estimation is exactly what it says: an estimate. It is a way of projecting efficacy of risk reduction without waiting for years to demonstrate efficacy (or a lack of it).

Appraising the health of a community can also be a source of civic pride if the appraisal is good, or a spur to action if it is not. It is easy to imagine; communities bidding for new industries on the grounds of a demonstrably healthy workforce. It is also easy to imagine the new industry listening to the argument, because we already know that a healthier workforce is a cheaper workforce. Risk estimation can also be a useful means of needs assessment for program development, for public relations, or for policy decisions. It provides a tool for simulating the results of any number of health policy options in terms of deaths postponed or diseases prevented.

Community risk estimation can be used for business purposes. For

*Director of Research, Lifespan Research Institute, Englewood, Florida

Reprinted with the permission of Harriet H. Imrey, Ph.D., Lifespan Institute, Englewood, Florida, and the Society of Prospective Medicine. This paper appeared in the *Proceedings of the 21st Annual Meeting of the Society of Prospective Medicine*; 1986 (Pp. 8–11).

instance, in the public health "business," we will hear a description later in this meeting of an enormously clever and successful lobbying campaign for a larger health promotion budget in Michigan. Private vendors of health risk appraisal instruments have already discovered the marketing potential for cost-effectiveness projections following worksite wellness programs—in this case, the individual company is the community of interest.

Before giving you a choice of several methods for estimating community risk, I would like to review some of the reasons for approaching this issue carefully. The bottom line for risk estimation in the community is calculating the Population Attributable Risk Proportion (PARP)—the percentage of deaths due to a particular risk factor—then multiplying this percentage by the number of deaths in the community. The only parameters you need to calculate this figure are the proportion of the population with the risk factor and the relative risk of death or disease for people who have the factor compared to those who do not:

$$PARP = \frac{p(RR-1)}{1 + p(RR-1)}$$

This is very straightforward when you are working with one binary risk factor (people have it or they don't). The only complications arise when you want to use more than one risk factor or a risk factor with several gradients of risk—such as heavy smoking, light smoking, and nonsmoking. Unfortunately, we almost always want to do it this way, and have to cope with the complexities.

The simplest example is a dataset based on two risk factors, where the data show no confounding and no interaction. For our purposes, "no confounding" means that people who have or do not have risk factor A have equal probabilities of having risk factor B; A and B are not associated. "No interaction" means that the relative risk of B is the same whether or not the person has risk factor A. (See Table E-1).

The easiest way to look at Population Attributable Risk, when you have a complete set of data such as this, is to look at the death rate among the group which has neither risk factor, and see by what proportion the total death rate would go down if everybody were at that low risk level. In this case, it would be 42.86%. In the real world, we don't have this information for the community we are working with, so we have to make the first great leap of faith: we assume that a relative risk represents some sort of biological truth which applies to the world at large, and that unknown risk factors are not busily confounding our data source. Then we can go ahead and use these relative risk figures with prevalence data from our own community.

Again, back to the real world, we might not know anything about the joint distribution of the risk factors and know only what proportion of people have factor A and what proportion have factor B. In this case only, we have the option of working with one variable at a time. The total PARP, calculated by combining the PARP figures for the two variables and using the last formula for Table E-1, is the same as that calculated with the first formula. One important thing to notice here is that the PARP figures cannot be added together, because the same death would be accounted for more than once: your community risk estimate would look odd, if you promised to reduce the death rate by 150%.

The next example shows the effects of confounding: what happens when your risk factors are not distributed independently in the original data sources. (Table E-2) The important thing here is that the relative risks you would be using are not the true (unconfounded) relative risks: part of the effect measured for factor A is due to the larger proportion of B people in the A category, and vice versa. Both relative risks are overestimates of the true relative risk—i.e., the risk after adjustment for confounding. The result in this case is an overestimate of the community attributable risk by 18%.

Table E-3 shows confounding and interaction at the same time. If the only information you have is two separate relative risks and the population prevalence for each, your community attributable risk estimate will be inaccurate.

The point of this somewhat tedious review is to demonstrate that you will almost never have enough information to estimate community risk correctly for more than a very few variables at a time, because you need to be sure that the relative risks have been adjusted for confounding, that interactions have been accounted for, and that you know the joint distribution of all risk factors in your population. The latter procedure becomes especially tedious when more than a very few risk factors are involved.

The catch to this methodological warning is that these conditions cannot be met with relative risk data available at this point in time. The choices are to do nothing—even though many of us have a real need for estimates of community risk—or to proceed very carefully with the best data we can get, but make no unwarranted claims about the precision of the estimates. By supporting the use of individual health risk appraisals, we have already decided to take the latter course. All of us are barefoot empiricists who jump into applications based on epidemiologic evidence which usually falls far short of proof. What we do is make decisions on the weight of the evidence, as a jury in a civil court must do. If we waited for "beyond a reasonable doubt," we would still hesitate about advocating any form of health education or health promotion activities.

We have just reviewed the methodological reasons why community risk estimation should *not* be attempted. However, here are some directions to accomplish such an estimation. Table E–4 shows what to do if the only facts you know are the proportion of the population with each of several risk factors, and the relative risks which apply to that factor. You have to have faith that the risk factors are distributed independently in the study population the relative risks came from and in your own community, and faith that there is no interaction among the risk factors. Your leap of faith will be less strenuous if you don't try to account for factors you know to be related—such as relative weight, blood pressure, and exercise—in the same model. Nobody can force you to be sensible about it, because the equations don't care one way or the other. The Regional Health Resource Center has computer software geared to data from the state Risk Factor Prevalence Surveys, which will print out the number of postponable deaths following simulated changes in population prevalence. Even our program will fail to blow up if the user asks for non-independent risk factors.

You can do a much better job of community risk estimation if you know the joint prevalence distribution of all the risk factors in your model, and if you have faith that the relative risks you use are "pure" ones—i.e., relative risks adjusted for confounding or derived from a multivariate model. You might even have relative risks for interactions. In practice, if you know the joint prevalence of risk factors, you probably know the composite relative risk of each member of your community sample. You have a choice of equations. Table E–5 shows the computation of the population attributable risk proportion for grouped data. If you have a computerized dataset with risk factor prevalence survey data, it is more efficient to use this formula:

$$PARP = 1 - \frac{N}{\Sigma CRR}$$

The composite relative risk for a community (relative to what the community would be like if every resident reduced all reducible risk factors) is always the inverse of the population unattributable risk proportion, just as the composite relative risk for an individual is the inverse of his own unattributable risk proportion. Given this fact, it is easy to compare two states or communities directly, and make inappropriate comparisons. One can imagine health educators arguing indefinitely over a model which asserted that Montana is exactly 37.5% healthier than Arkansas. A large lawsuit over a suspected environmental contaminant is going to center on the argument, based on this methodology, that the cancer rate in the affected community, after accounting for other KNOWN risk factors, was even lower than the cancer rate in the control community, proving that no excess cases could be blamed on a carcinogen in the water supply.

In the future, we will see a growing number of examples of this sort, and can expect to see more people estimating community risk based on more accurate models. In the meantime, it is necessary to be very cautious about creating synthetic models from very crude data, but that doesn't mean it can't be done. We haven't even touched on questions of selecting all-cause mortality models versus summing over individual causes of death, although the former is generally more conservative. We also haven't considered inaccuracies based upon different risk factor prevalence distributions in different age groups: the safest procedure is to use proportions and relative risks for the narrowest age groups for which data are available. We haven't talked about additive versus multiplicative models, although similar techniques have been derived for additive models. Failing to consider any one of these issues can make your community risk estimates less accurate. However, if you back off because the procedure is complicated, you will miss the opportunity to get some very interesting and useful information which may be only a little bit in error.

In summary, take whatever information you have, add any information you can reasonbly get, and take full advantage of every single piece of it. If you have access to your state's Risk Factor Prevalence Survey database, or to a file of computerized health risk appraisals, you are ready to do community risk appraisal with a fair degree of accuracy for a very small investment.

Technical Notation: How to Read the Tables.

The probability notation used in the examples may be unfamiliar to many readers, but is not nearly so complicated as it looks. The A and B stand for two different risk factors, such as smoking and obesity. A bar over the top is a negative symbol: it means that the risk factor is not present. In Table E-1, the second row that starts out with $A\bar{B}$ stands for that part of the population of 10,000 people who have risk factor A (they smoke), but do not have risk factor B (they are not overweight). The number (N) of people in that category is 3,000; the category's proportion (p) of the total is .30. The rate (r) of death is .02, meaning that $3000 \times .02 = 60$ people in the category will die (d). The relative risk (RR) is the death rate in that category compared to the death rate among people who do not have either of the risk factors (the row that starts with $\bar{A}\bar{B}$), so the relative risk for category $A\bar{B}$ is $.02/.01 = 2$. It takes a little bit of time to figure out any new notation, but using this one can be very time-saving when communicating complex numerical examples.

Table E-1. *PARP Example of Two Risk Factors with No Confounding and No Interaction*

	N	p	r	d	RR
A B	1000	.10	.04	40	4.0
A $\bar{\text{B}}$	3000	.30	.02	60	2.0
$\bar{\text{A}}$ B	1500	.15	.02	30	2.0
$\bar{\text{A}}$ $\bar{\text{B}}$	4500	.45	.01	45	1.0
TOTAL	10,000		.0175	175	

$$\text{Population Attributable Risk Proportion (PARP)} = \frac{r(TOTAL) - r(\bar{A}\,\bar{B})}{r(TOTAL)} =$$

$$= \frac{.0175 - .01}{.0175} = 42.86\%$$

OR

$$1 - \frac{1}{\Sigma pRR} = 1 - \frac{1}{.10(4) + .30(2) + .15(2) + .45(1)} = 1 - \frac{1}{1.75} = 42.86\%$$

One variable at a time:

	N	p	r	d	RR
A	4000	.40	.025	100	2.0
$\bar{\text{A}}$	6000	.60	.0125	75	1.0
	10,000		.0175	175	

PARP(A) = 28.57%

	N	p	r	d	RR
B	2500	.25	.028	70	2.0
$\bar{\text{B}}$	7500	.75	.014	105	1.0
	10,000		.0175	175	

PARP(B) = 20.0%

TOTAL Population Attributable Risk Proportion = $1 - \pi\,(1 - PARP(X)) =$

$$1 - (1 - 28.57\%)(1 - 20.0\%) = 42.86\%$$

(Note: See Technical Notation for commentary on the notations used in the tables)

Table E-2. *PARP Example of Two Risk Factors with Confounding and No Interaction (P(BIA) = .15, not .10)*

Confounding: the likelihood of possessing risk factor B is different depending on whether or not the person possesses factor A; i.e., a sedentary person may be somewhat more likely to smoke than a jogger.

	N	p	r	d	RR
A B	1500	.15	.04	60	4.0
A $\bar{B}$	2500	.25	.02	50	2.0
$\bar{A}$ B	1000	.10	.02	20	2.0
$\bar{A}$ $\bar{B}$	5000	.50	.01	50	1.0
	10000		.018	180	

$$PARP = \frac{.018 - .01}{.018} = 44.44\%$$

One variable at a time:

	N	p	r	d	RR
A	4000	.40	.0275	110	2.36
$\bar{A}$	6000	.60	.0117	70	1.0
	10000		.018	180	

PARP(A) = 35.0%

	N	p	r	d	RR
B	2500	.25	.0320	80	2.41
$\bar{B}$	7500	.75	.0133	100	1.0
	10000		.0180	180	

PARP(B) = 26.06%

$$1 - (1-.35)(1-.2606) = 51.94\% \text{ (NOT RIGHT)}$$

Table E-3. *PARP Example of Two Risk Factors with Confounding and Interaction (RR(AB)* = 5, not 4)

Interaction: The effect on mortality of risk factor B is greater if the person also possesses risk factor A; i.e., a sedentary lifestyle may be more hazardous among smokers than among nonsmokers.

	N	p	r	d	RR
A B	1500	.15	.05	75	5.0
A $\bar{\text{B}}$	2500	.25	.02	50	2.0
$\bar{\text{A}}$ B	1000	.10	.02	20	2.0
$\bar{\text{A}}$ $\bar{\text{B}}$	5000	.50	.01	50	1.0
	10000		.0195	195	

$$\text{PARP} = \frac{.0195 - .01}{.0195} = 48.72\%$$

One variable at a time:

	N	p	r	d	RR
A	4000	.40	.03125	125	2.68
$\bar{\text{A}}$	6000	.60	.0117	70	1.0
	10000		.0195	195	

PARP = 40.2%

	N	p	r	d	RR
B	2500	.25	.038	95	2.85
$\bar{\text{B}}$	7500	.75	.0133	100	1.0
	10000		.0195	195	

PARP = 31.62%

$$1 - (1-.402)(1-.3162) = 59.11\% \text{ (NOT RIGHT)}$$

Table E-4. *Risk Estimation Process with Community Prevalence Rates for Individual Risk Factors*

WHAT YOU KNOW:

1) Number (or rate) of deaths
2) Relative risks (RR) for one or more risk factors
3) Community prevalence rates (p) for one or more risk factors.

WHAT YOU BELIEVE:

Risk factors are distributed independently in the population and there are no interactions among the relative risks.

188 *NEEDS ASSESSMENT STRATEGIES*

WHAT YOU DO:

1) For ONE risk factor:

$$PARP = \frac{p(RR-1)}{1 + p(RR-1)}$$

Deaths which may be postponable = # of deaths × PARP

2) For ONE or MORE risk factors:

$$PARP = 1 - \pi \ (1 - PARP(X))$$

i.e., if the PARP for smoking is 30% and the PARP for inactivity is 20%, the total attributable risk proportion is 1 — (1–.30) (1–.20) = 44%

Table E-5. *Risk Estimation Process with Community Prevalence Rates for Combinations of Risk Factors*

WHAT YOU KNOW:

1) Number (or rate) of deaths
2) Relative risks (RR) for one or more risk factors
3) Community prevalence rates (p) for each combination of risk factors, from a population survey or from risk appraisals

WHAT YOU BELIEVE:

The risk factors are not distributed independently, but you believe that the relative risks in your model do not interact with one another except in those cases where you have identified a separate relative risk for the categories where interactions take place.

WHAT YOU DO:

$$PARP = 1 - \frac{1}{\Sigma pCRR}$$

Where p is the proportion of the population with a particular combination of risk factors, and CRR is the composite relative risk for that particular combination (i.e., the product of all of the relative risks for each separate risk factor)

Table E-6. *Risk Estimation Process with Risk Factor Prevalence Data for Each Subject*

WHAT YOU KNOW:

1) Number (or rate) of deaths
2) Relative risks (RR) for one or more risk factors
3) Risk factor prevalence data for each individual in your population sample

WHAT YOU BELIEVE:

The relative risks in your model do not interact with one another except in those cases where you have a separate relative risk for the categories where interactions take place.

WHAT YOU DO:

$$PARP = 1 - \frac{1}{\Sigma CRR}$$

Where CRR is the Composite Relative Risk (product of individual relative risks) for each individual in your sample of N people.

BIBLIOGRAPHY

Abbey, D.E. "Worksite Wellness Using the CDC Health Risk Appraisal (Adaption, Implementation, and Evaluation)." In *Proceedings of the 21st Annual Meeting of the Society of Prospective Medicine: Equipping the Professional/Protecting the Consumer.* Indianapolis: Society of Prospective Medicine, Publishers, 1986; 46-48.

Abramson, J.H. *Survey Methods in Community Medicine.* New York: Churchill-Livingstone Publishers, 1979.

Agor, W.H. *Intuitive Management.* Englewood Cliffs, NJ: Prentice Hall, Inc.; 1984.

American Cancer Society. *TSE Guidelines.* Virginia Division; 1982.

American Cancer Society. *Testicular Self-Examination.* Milwaukee District, Wisconsin Division; 1986.

American Cancer Society. *Cancer Facts and Figures: 1988.* Atlanta, GA; 1988.

Amler, R.W. "Documentation of Preventable Morbidity and Mortality: The Carter Center Health Consultation and Adult Health Risk Appraisal Project." In *Proceedings of the 21st Annual Meeting of the Society of Prospective Medicine: Equipped the Professional/Protecting the Consumer.* Indianapolis: Society of Prospective Medicine, Publishers; 1986; 4-5.

Amler, R.W. Interim Report: *Health Risk Appraisal.* Atlanta, GA: The Carter Center, Emery University; 1987.

Antilla, S. and H. Sender. "Getting Consumers in Focus." *Dunn's Business Month.* 119: 78-80; 1982.

Axworthy, L., Grant, M., Cassidy, J., and G. Siamandas. *Meeting the Problems and Needs of Resident Advisory Groups.* Winnipeg: The Institute of Urban Studies; 1973.

Bailey, A.R. "Who Should Set Health Priorities?" *Journal of Extension.* 11: 20-27; 1973.

Baker, E., Levenstein, C., and M.C. White. "Worksite Health Promotion Utilizing Health Risk Appraisal: The Painters Project." In *Proceedings of the 21st Annual Meeting of the Society of Prospective Medicine: Equipping the Professional/Protecting the Consumer.* Indianapolis: Society of Prospective Medicine, Publishers, 1986; 31-36.

Bates, I.J., and A.E. Winder. *Introduction to Health Education.* Palo Alto, CA: Mayfield Publishing Company; 1984.

Beery, W., Schoenbach, V.J., and E.H. Wagner. *Health Risk Appraisal: Methods and Programs, with Annotated Bibliography.* Rockville, MD: U.S. Department of Health and Human Services, National Center for Health Services Research and Health Care Technology Assessment; 1986.

Bellenger, D.N., Bernhardt, K.L., and J.L. Goldstucker. *Qualitative Research in Marketing.* Chicago: American Marketing Association; 1976.

Bernstein, D. "Focus Group Rapport Can Mislead." *Advertising Age.* 49: 50; July 10, 1978.

Blesch, K.S. "Health Beliefs about Testicular Cancer and Self-Examination among Professional Men." *Oncology Nursing Forum.* 16: 29-33; 1986.

Boyd, H. W., Westfall, R., and S. T. Starch. *Marketing Research Text and Case.* Homewood, Illinois: Richard D. Irwin, Inc.; 1981.

Breslow, L., Fielding, J., Afifi, A.A., Coulson, A., Kheifets, L., Valdiviezo, N., Goetz, A., McTyre, R., Peterson, K. and K. Dane. *Risk Factor Update Project: Final Report.* Atlanta, GA: U.S. Department of Health and Human Services, Centers for Disease Control, Center for Health Promotion and Education; 1985.

Briggs Myers, I. *Gifts Differing.* Palo Alto, CA: Consulting Psychologists Press, Inc.; 1980.

Centers for Disease Control. *Interpretation of the Health Risk Appraisal Printout.* Atlanta, Georgia: U.S. Department of Health Human Services; 1984.

Churchill, G. *Marketing Research: Methodological Foundations.* Hinsdale, Illinois: Dryden Press; 1979.

Delbecq, A.L., Van de Ven, A.H., and D.H. Gustafson. *Group Techniques for Program Planning.* Glenview, Illinois: Scott, Foresman, and Company; 1975.

191

Dever, G.E.A. *Community Health Analysis: A Holistic Approach.* Rockville, Maryland: Aspen Systems; 1980.

Dever, G.E.A. *Epidemiology in Health Services Management.* Rockville, MD: Aspen Systems Corporation; 1984.

Dillman, D.D. *Mail and Telephone Surveys: The Total Design Method.* New York: John Wiley and Sons, Inc.; 1978.

Dorsay, R.H., Cuneo, W.D., Somkin, C.P. and I.S. Tekawa. "Breast Self-Examination: Improving Competence and Frequency in a Classroom Setting." *American Journal of Public Health.* 78: 520-522; 1988.

Edington, D.W. and L. Yen. "Worksite Health Promotion Utilizing Health Risk Appraisal." In *Proceedings of the 21st Annual Meeting of the Society of Prospective Medicine: Equipping the Professional/Protecting the Consumer.* Indianapolis: Society of Prospective Medicine, Publishers; 1986; 37-39.

Erdos, P.N. *Professional Mail Surveys.* Malabar, Florida: Robert E. Krieger Publishing Company; 1983.

Foster, R.S., and M.C. Costanza. "Breast Self-Examination Practices and Breast Cancer Survival." *Cancer.* 53: 999-1005; 1984.

Foxman, B., and D.W. Edington. "The Accuracy of Health Risk Appraisal in Predicting Mortality." *American Journal of Public Health.* 77: 971-974; 1987.

Frank, I.N., Keys, H.M., and C.S. McCune. "Urologic and Male Genital Cancers." In P. Rubin (ed.) *Clinical Oncology.* New York: American Cancer Society; 1983.

Frey, J.H. *Survey Research by Telephone.* Beverly Hills, CA: Sage Publications; 1983.

Gage, T.J. "Theories Differ on Use of Focus Group." *Advertising Age.* 51: 519-522; 1980.

Gilmore, G.D. "Needs Assessment Processes for Community Health Education." *International Journal of Health Education.* 20: 164-173; 1977.

Gilmore, G.D. "Planning For Family Wellness." *Health Education.* 10: 12-16; 1979.

Gilmore, G.D., Dosch, M.F., and T.L. Hood. "The Development, Implementation and Evaluation of the La Crosse Wellness Project." Presented at the 19th meeting of The Society of Prospective Medicine, Atlanta, GA; 1983.

Gilmore, G.D., Dosch, M.F., and T.L. Hood. "Continuing Evaluation of the La Crosse Wellness Project: Longitudinal and Community-Based Process and Impact Analyses." In *Proceedings of the 20th Annual Meeting of the Society of Prospective Medicine: A Decade of Survival, Past, Present, Future.* Washington, D.C.: Society of Prospective Medicine, Publishers; 1985; 82-85.

Gorden, R.L. *Interviewing: Strategy, Techniques, and Tactics.* Chicago: The Dorsey Press; 1987.

Green, L.W., and F.M. Lewis. *Measurement and Evaluation in Health Education and Health Promotion.* Palo Alto, CA: Mayfield Publishing Company; 1986.

Green, L.W., Kreuter, M.W., Deeds, S.G., and K.B. Partridge. *Health Education Planning: A Diagnostic Approach.* Palo Alto, CA: Mayfield Publishing Company; 1980.

Hall, J.H., and J.D. Zwemer. *Prospective Medicine.* Indianapolis: Methodist Hospital of Indiana; 1979.

Hanson, P., Matheson, G., and P.A. Reed. "A Tri-County Needs Assessment for the Purpose of Rural Health Promotion Program Development." *Home Health Care Nurse.* 1: 22-27; 1983.

Health Information Center. *Healthfinder: Health Risk Appraisals.* Washington, D.C.: U.S. Department of Health and Human Services, Office of Disease Prevention and Health Promotion; 1987.

"How To Use the Key Informant Survey Technique." *How To: Evaluate Education Programs.* 1-6; February, 1985.

Hyer, G.C. and C.L. Melby. "Health Risk Appraisals: Use and Misuse." *Family and Community Health.* 8: 13-25; 1985.

Johansen, R., Vallee, J., and K. Spangler. *Electronic Meetings: Technical Alternatives and Social Choices*. Reading, Massachusetts: Addison-Wesley Publishing Company, 1979.

Imrey, H.H. "Community Risk Estimation." In *Proceedings of the 21st Annual Meeting of the Society of Prospective Medicine: Equipping the Professional/Protecting the Consumer*. Indianapolis: Society of Prospective Medicine, Publishers; 1986; 8-11.

Keller, K.L., Sliepcevich, E.M., Vitello, E.M., Lacey, E.P., and W.R. Wright. "Assessing Beliefs About and Needs of Senior Citizens Using the Focus Group Interview: A Qualitative Approach." *Health Education.* 18: 44-49; 1987.

Kimmel, W. *Needs Assessment: A Critical Perspective*. Washington, D.C.: Office of Program Systems, Department of Health, Education, and Welfare; 1977.

Linstone, H. and M. Turoff (eds.). *The Delphi Method: Techniques and Applications*. New York: Addison-Wesley Publishing Company, Inc.; 1975.

Luck, D.J., Wales, H.G., Taylor, D.A., and R.S. Rubin. *Market Research*. Englewood Cliffs, New Jersey: Prentice Hall, Inc.; 1982.

Lund, B. and S. McGechaen. *Continuing Education Programmer's Manual*. Victoria, British Columbia: Continuing Education Division, Ministry of Education; 1981.

Luther, S.L., Sroka, S., Goormastic, M., and J.E. Montie. "Teaching Breast and Testicular Self-Exams: Evaluation of a High School Curriculum Pilot Project." *Health Education.* 16: 40-43; 1985.

Marciano, L.A. "Prevalence of Risk Factors Among Teens." In *Proceedings of the 21st Annual Meeting of the Society of Prospective Medicine: Equipping the Professional/Protecting the Consumer*. Indianapolis: Society of Prospective Medicine, Publishers. 1986; 14-15.

Matthews, M.E., Mahaffey, M.J., Lerner, R.N., and W.L. Bunch. "Profiles of the Future for Administrative Dieticians via the Delphi Technique." *Journal of the American Dietetic Association.* 66: 494-499; 1975.

McKillip, J. *Need Analysis: Tools for the Human Services and Education*. Beverly Hills, CA: Sage Publications; 1987.

Miskovic, D. "Behind the Mirror: Here are Some Rules that can Help Sharpen the Value of Focus Groups." *Advertising Age.* 51: 55; 1980.

Moriarty, D.G. "Health Risk Appraisal for Underserved Publications: An Overview." In *Proceedings of the 21st Annual Meeting of the Society of Prospective Medicine: Equipping the Professional/Protecting the Consumer*. Indianapolis: Society of Prospective Medicine, publishers. 1986; 49.

Noack, H. "Concepts of Health and Health Promotion." in Abelin, T., Brzezinski, Z.J., and V.D.L. Carstairs (eds.) *Measurement in Health Promotion and Protection*. Geneva: World Health Organization; 1987.

O'Malley, M.S., and S.W. Fletcher. "Screening for Breast Cancer with Breast Self-Examination: A Critical Review." *JAMA.* 257: 2197-2203; 1987.

Poole, M.S., and R.Y. Hirokawa. "Communication and Group Decision-Making: A Critical Assessment." In Hirokawa, R.Y., and M.S. Poole (eds.) *Communication and Group Decision-Making*. Beverly Hills, CA: Sage Publications; 1986.

Public Health Service. *Healthy People: The Surgeon General's Report on Health Promotion and Disease Prevention*. Washington, D.C.: U.S. Department of Health, Education, and Welfare; 1979.

Rice, R.E., and G. Love. "Electronic Emotion: Socioemotional Content in a Computer-Mediated Communication Network." *Communication Research.* 14: 85-108; 1987.

Richards, M.J.S., and S.L. Inhorn. *1988 Breast Cancer Detection Awareness Project Update*. Madison, WI: American Cancer Society, Wisconsin Division; 1988.

Richardson, A., and C. Bray. *Promoting Health Through Participation*. London: Policy Studies Institute; 1987.

Richardson, G.E. "Health Risk Versus Lifestyle Improvement Instruments." In *Proceedings of* the 21st Annual Meeting of the Society of Prospective Medicine: Equipping the Profesisonal/Protecting the Consumer. Indianapolis: Society of Prospective Medicine, Publishers. 1986; 59-61.

Robbins, L.C., and J.H. Hall. *How to Practice Prospective Medicine*. Indianapolis: Methodist Hospital of Indiana; 1979.

Ross, H.S., and P.R. Mico. *Theory and Practice in Health Education*. Palo Alto, CA: Mayfield Publishing Company; 1980.

Rowley, D., Mills, S., Kellum, C., and B. Avery. "Are Current Health Risk Appraisals Suitable for Black Women?" In *Proceedings of the 21st Annual Meeting of the Society of Prospective Medicine: Equipping the Professional/Protecting the Consumer*. Indianapolis: Society of Prospective Medicine, Publishers. 1986; 50-53.

Sacks, J.J., Krushat, W.M., and J. Newman. "Reliability of the Health Hazard Appraisal." *American Journal of Public Health*. 70: 730-732; 1980.

Safer, M.A. "An Evaluation of the Health Hazard Appraisal Based on Survey Data from a Randomly Selected Publication." *Public Health Reports*. 97: 31-37; 1982.

Schottenfeld, D., Warshauer, M.E., Sherlock, S., Zauber, A.G., LeDer, M., and R. Payne. "The Epidemiology of Testicular Cancer in Young Adults." *American Journal of Epidemiology*. 112: 232-246; 1980.

Scott, D.H. and R.M. Cabral. "Predicting Hazardous Lifestyles Among Adolescents Based on Health-Risk Assessment Data." *American Journal of Health Promotion*. 2:23-28; 1988.

Shy, C.M., Rowland, A., Ramsey, D., and M. McLanahan. "Project to Modify the CDC Health Risk Appraisal for Blue Collar Workers." In *Proceedings of the 21st Annual Meeting of the Society of Prospective Medicine: Equipping the Professional/Protecting the Consumer*. Indianapolis: Society of Prospective Medicine, Publishers. 1986; 40-43.

Smith, K.W., McKinlay, S.M., and B.D. Thorington. "The Validity of Health Risk Appraisal Instruments for Assessing Coronary Heart Disease Risk." *American Journal of Public Health*. 77: 419-424; 1987.

Sork, T.J. "Determining Priorities." Vancouver, British Columbia: University of British Columbia; 1982.

Sudman, S., and N.M. Bradburn. *Asking Questions: A Practical Guide to Questionnaire Design*. San Francisco: Jossey-Bass Publishers; 1983.

Stewart, D.W. *Secondary Research: Information, Sources and Methods*. Beverly Hills, CA: Sage Publications; 1984.

Trecker, H.B., and A.R. Trecker. *Working with Groups, Committees, and Communities*. Chicago: Follett Publishing Company; 1979.

U.S. Health Resources Administration. *Educating the Public About Health: A Planning Guide*. Rockville, MD: Department of Health, Education, and Welfare; 1977.

Van de Ven, A.H., and A.L. Delbecq. "Nominal Versus Interacting Group Processes for Committee Decision-Making Effectiveness." *Academy of Management Journal*. 14: 203-212; 1971.

Vickery, D.M., and J.F. Fries. *Take Care of Yourself: A Consumer's Guide to Medical Care*. Reading, Massachusetts: Addison-Wesley Publishing Company; 1977.

Webb, E.J., Campbell, D.T., Schwartz, R.D., and L. Sechrest. *Unobtrusive Measures: Nonreactive Research in the Social Sciences*. Chicago: Rand McNally and Company, 1966.

Webb, E.J., and K.E. Weick. "Unobtrusive Measures in Organizational Theory." In J. Van Maanen (ed.) *Qualitative Methodology*: 209-224. Beverly Hills: Sage Publications, 1983.

Williams, R.T. A Model for Identifying Mental Health Education Needs. Madison, WI: University of Wisconsin; Doctoral Dissertation; 1978.

Witkin, B.R. *Assessing Needs in Educational and Social Programs*. San Francisco: Jossey-Bass Publishers; 1984.

Working Group on Concepts and Principles of Health Promotion. "Health Promotion: Concepts and Principles." In Abelin, T., Brzezinski, Z.J., and V.D.L. Carstairs (eds.) *Measurement in Health Promotion and Protection*. Geneva: World Health Organization; 1987.

World Health Organization. *Health Education: A Programme Review*. Geneva; 1974.
World Health Organization. *Basic Documents*. Geneva; 1985.
Yankauer, A. "New to the Journal from NCHS." *American Journal of Public Health*. 77: 1502; 1987.
Zikmund, W.G. *Exploring Marketing Research*. Chicago: Dryden Press; 1982.

Index

Author Index

Subject Index